Death by Appointment

Death by Appointment:

A Rational Guide to the Assisted Dying Debate

By

Ilora Finlay and Robert Preston

Cambridge Scholars Publishing

Death by Appointment: A Rational Guide to the Assisted Dying Debate

By Ilora Finlay and Robert Preston

This book first published 2020

Cambridge Scholars Publishing

Lady Stephenson Library, Newcastle upon Tyne, NE6 2PA, UK

British Library Cataloguing in Publication Data
A catalogue record for this book is available from the British Library

ISBN (10): 1-5275-5978-5
ISBN (13): 978-1-5275-5978-3

CONTENTS

INTRODUCTION

At 9-45am on 11 September 2015 Rob Marris, at the time MP for Wolverhampton South West, rose to his feet in the House of Commons to introduce his Assisted Dying No.2 Bill. It was designated 'No. 2' because there was another, almost identical, Private Member bill in the House of Lords at the same time in the name of Lord Falconer of Thoroton: it had been tabled a week or so before Mr Marris's bill.

Unusually for a Friday, the Chamber was crowded for Mr Marris's presentation of his bill. After he had resumed his seat, a large number of MPs spoke, sometimes with passion, for or against the bill. Shortly after 2pm a Division was called. 118 MPs voted to support the bill, 330 voted to reject it. The bill fell as a result.

Mr Marris's attempt to change the law was not the first of its kind. Between 2003 and 2005 Lord Joffe had tabled three similar Private Member bills in the House of Lords. None of them had made progress and in May 2006 the last one was put to a vote in the Chamber and rejected by 148 votes to 100. In 2013 and 2014 Lord Falconer had introduced similar bills, the second of which reached its committee stage but progressed no further. As we write, Lord Falconer has tabled yet another 'assisted dying' bill in the 2020-21 session of Parliament.

However, Parliament has done more than consider a succession of 'assisted dying' bills. In 2004, in response to the second of Lord Joffe's three Private Member bills a select committee of Peers was established to examine the subject in depth under the chairmanship of Lord Mackay of Clashfern, who had been Lord Chancellor from 1987 to 1997.

The committee took its work very seriously. In the nine months between its first meeting and its report it cross-examined over 140 witnesses, many of whom were experts in fields such as medicine, the law, mental health and ethics. It gathered some of this evidence via visits to three overseas jurisdictions - the US State of Oregon, The Netherlands and Switzerland - where 'assisted dying' in one form or another had been legalised. It also invited members of the public to write in with their views. The response was over 12,000 emails or letters. Some of them were brief statements of support for or opposition to a change in the law: others were longer commentaries on specific aspects of the subject. The committee's three-volume report, when it was published in April 2005, ran to nearly a thousand pages. It is probably fair to say that it has been the most comprehensive examination of this subject in Britain to date.

In our view the evidence received by the committee raised serious doubts about whether 'assisted dying' should be legalised. However, opinion within the committee was divided on the question and its report summarised the evidence received on both sides and presented a balanced analysis of the issues. Although the political debate on 'assisted dying' has continued since the report was published, much of its content and analysis remains relevant today and we have referred to it in a number of places in the chapters which follow [1] . It is a document which any serious student of 'assisted dying' would be well advised to study.

This book is written for those who wish to try and find a way through the thickets of this complex and emotive subject and who are interested in seeing the arguments analysed and examined. What we have tried to do is to provide a birds-eye view of the

---

[1] Contains Parliamentary information licensed under the Open Parliament Licence v3.0 https://www.parliament.uk/site-information/copyright-parliament/open-parliament-licence/

subject and to show how the various parts interact with each other.

There are respectable arguments to be heard on both sides of the 'assisted dying' debate. Our assessment, after careful examination of the evidence, is that the law should not be changed, and certainly not on the terms which have been proposed. But we respect the sincerity of those who take a different view.

Our aim in the chapters which follow has been to elucidate the main components of this complex debate – the law, medical practice, end-of-life care, ethics, safeguarding and the experience of those jurisdictions overseas that have gone down the 'assisted dying' road. We have examined a variety of arguments put forward for legalisation and explained why we conclude that they do not justify changing the law. We have endeavoured throughout to do so respectfully and recognising that this is an issue that can generate deeply-held emotions.

Having read what we have written, readers must make up their own minds as to whether the law should be changed. If this book has prompted some to stop and think, it will have achieved its purpose.

CHAPTER ONE

ASSISTED DYING AND THE LAW

ROBERT PRESTON

"It is a hugely compassionate case and I would do exactly as the policeman did...But I would not expect the law to be changed to allow that"

The Policeman's Dilemma

The date is 13 January 2005. A select committee of the House of Lords is hearing evidence on a Private Member's Bill - Lord Joffe's Assisted Dying for the Terminally Ill Bill, which had been tabled the year before. The committee has already spent four months taking evidence, not just in Britain but also in the US State of Oregon and in Holland. And a week or two later it will go to Switzerland.

On that day the committee has before it a panel of people drawn from different religious faiths - an Anglican theologian, a Catholic bishop, a rabbi and a Muslim doctor. One of the members of the committee puts a question to them. He describes a situation that is sometimes known as 'the policeman's dilemma'. Here is what he says, taken from the official transcript of evidence:

> *"It was the case in the United States where a driver was trapped in a burning lorry. There was no possibility of extricating him and he was about to be burned to death and suffer a very painful end. A*

> *policeman was on the scene and he asked the policeman 'Will you shoot me?' and the policeman did"*[1].

The panel of witnesses were asked whether they believed the policeman's action was morally justifiable. The same question had been put to other witnesses on other occasions. Everyone who had been asked had found the question difficult to answer. If they had had answered 'No, the policeman was wrong to shoot the man', they could be accused of heartlessness. On the other hand, if they had answered 'Yes, he did the right thing', they invited the riposte that in that case they would agree with legalised euthanasia.

On this occasion one of the witnesses gave a response which might not have been expected from a man of the cloth. "*It is a hugely compassionate case*", he said, "*and I would do exactly as the policeman did and I hope you would too*"

Then he added:

> "*but I would not expect the law to be changed to allow that*"[2].

This exchange, it seems to me, goes to the heart of the political debate about what is being called 'assisted dying'. The central question is not whether such actions are morally right or wrong or whether or not they are a compassionate thing to do. It is about whether they should be licensed by law.

It is one thing to say that an illegal act performed in exceptional circumstances is understandable, that we can empathise with it and that it should not be prosecuted, but quite another to say that permission should be given in advance for such acts to be performed in specified circumstances. No one, for example, would want to see a parent prosecuted for breaking the speed limit while rushing a desperately sick child to hospital. No one would want to see the full force of the law brought to bear on a mother if she

---

[1] House of Lords Report 86-II (Session 2004-05), Page 495
[2] Ibid

stole out of desperation to feed her starving children. None of us would want to see a man prosecuted for assault if he inflicted injury on a nocturnal intruder while protecting his family. Yet who would seriously suggest that the law should be changed to license dangerous driving or theft or assault in advance and in prescribed circumstances? It is hard to believe anyone would. We expect the laws prohibiting such acts to be maintained to protect us all and we look to see exceptional cases dealt with exceptionally. That is what happens under current law with 'assisted dying'.

This is not to say that changes should never be made to existing laws. If it can be shown clearly that a law is unduly oppressive or that it is not fulfilling its purpose, fair and good. Let us look, therefore, at the law on 'assisted dying' and see whether or not this is the case.

What does the law say?

We need to begin by defining our terms. The term 'assisted dying' has no meaning in law. It is an artificial term, a euphemism coined by campaigners for legal change, meaning the supplying of lethal drugs by a doctor to a terminally patient who requests them and is thought to meet certain criteria. In law that is assisting suicide. In what follows, therefore, when I use the term 'assisted dying', I place the words in inverted commas.

The law differs slightly between England and Wales on the one hand and Scotland on the other. The law in Northern Ireland is, for all practical purposes, the same as the law in England and Wales, so I will not deal with it separately.

England and Wales

The law in question is the Suicide Act of 1961. Until then suicide had been a criminal offence and a person who attempted to commit suicide but survived could be prosecuted. The 1961 Act did not legalise suicide. It decriminalised it, meaning that charges would no longer be brought against anyone who attempted suicide. The distinction is an important one. Legalisation of an act implies that the act in question is seen as acceptable. Parliament was assured, however, during the passage of the Suicide Bill in 1961 that this was not the case with decriminalisation. The Home Office Minister moving the Bill's Third Reading stated that:

> *"Because we have taken the view, as Parliament and the Government have taken, that the treatment of people who attempt to commit suicide should no longer be through the criminal courts, it in no way lessens, nor should it lessen, the respect for the sanctity of life which we all share. It must not be thought that because we are changing the method of treatment for those unfortunate people, we seek to depreciate the gravity of the action of anyone who tries to commit suicide"*[3].

and that:

> *"I should like to state as solemnly as I can...that we wish to give no encouragement whatever to suicide"*[4].

Decriminalisation of suicide was accompanied in the 1961 Act by a provision (Clause 2) which made it unlawful to 'aid, abet, counsel or procure' the suicide or attempted suicide of another person. In other words, you would not be prosecuted if you attempted to take your own life but that did not mean you were free to help other people to take theirs. The wording of this provision was amended in 2009[5] and the offence broadened to one of 'encouraging or assisting' suicide in an attempt to counter encouragement of suicide by internet websites, a situation that could not have been foreseen in 1961.

---

[3] House of Commons Hansard, 28 July 1961, Cols 822-823

[4] House of Commons Hansard, 19 July 1961 Cols 1425-1426

[5] Coroners and Justice Act 2009, Clause 59

Scotland

The legal position is less clearly defined in Scotland than in England and Wales. In Scotland there is no statutory offence of assisting suicide - that is to say, there is no equivalent of Clause 2 of the 1961 Suicide Act. Assisting suicide is governed by the common law relating to homicide and could attract a charge of either murder or culpable homicide depending on whether there was evidence of a 'wicked intent to kill'. According to a committee of the Scottish Parliament which recently examined a Private Member's Bill to legalise assisted suicide, a charge of culpable homicide would be likely to be brought[6].

Prosecutorial Discretion

In England and Wales anyone found guilty by a court of encouraging or assisting another person's suicide is liable to a sentence of imprisonment for up to 14 years. At first sight this may look like a draconian penalty for someone who has helped a suffering loved one out of this world. But it is important to remember that it is a maximum sentence and that it does not oblige a court to impose a sentence of imprisonment at all - or, indeed, the Crown Prosecution Service to undertake a prosecution. Here we come to a very important feature of the law - prosecutorial discretion.

The 1961 Act included a provision that no prosecution may be undertaken without the consent of the Director of Public Prosecutions (DPP). When Parliament made this provision nearly 60 years ago, it recognised that helping someone to take his or her own life could cover a wide range of criminality. It could, at one end of the spectrum, be compassionate assistance given reluctantly, after much soul-searching and in response to earnest pleading in the

---

[6] 6th Report 2015 (Session 4): Stage 1 Report on Assisted Suicide (Scotland) Bill, Paragraph 27

face of severe suffering. At the other end of the scale, it could be malicious assistance motivated by personal gain and accompanied by pressure or abuse. The 1961 Act therefore requires the DPP to examine carefully the circumstances of any instance of assisting suicide and to reach a judgement of whether in that specific case a prosecution is in the public interest.

There is nothing unusual about this. In 1951 the then Attorney-General, Sir Hartley Shawcross, stated that *'it has never been the rule in this country – I hope it never will be – that suspected criminal offences must automatically be the subject of prosecution'*. The role of the DPP, he said, was to prosecute *'wherever it appears that the offence or the circumstances of its commission is or are of such a character that a prosecution in respect thereof is required in the public interest'*[7].

More recently, Sir Keir Starmer QC, MP, who held the office of DPP from 2008 to 2013, put it this way to Lord Falconer's Commission on Assisted Dying:

> *"There is a residual discretion for all offences whether to prosecute or not. This is a particular version of it. But it's not unique by any stretch of the imagination; it's the way our law operates*[8]"

In other words, deciding whether or not to prosecute is not just a matter of establishing whether the law has been broken - ie whether there has been illegality. That is part of it, of course. But it is also necessary to consider, if there has been a breach of the law, in what circumstances the offence was committed - ie what degree of criminality was involved. The same duality can be seen in the moral as well as in the legal field. As we have observed in the example of 'the policeman's dilemma', an act may be in itself morally reprehensible but the circumstances in which it was performed may be such that little or no guilt attaches to it.

[7] House of Commons Hansard, 29 January 1951, Col 681

[8] Commission on Assisted Dying, Oral Evidence 14 December 2010

In Scotland, though there is no specific offence of assisting suicide, a similar approach is adopted to south of the border. The Scottish Parliament was recently told by the Crown Office and Procurator Fiscal Service that cases of assisting suicide were "*very fact-sensitive*" and that "*under the current prosecution code prosecutors are encouraged to have regard to a wide range of factors when determining the potential criminality of conduct, including the motive for the behaviour*"[9].

Does it work?

So much for the system. Does it work? Assisting suicide is a very rare offence: on average, less than 20 cases throughout the whole of England and Wales cross the desk of the DPP in a year. By any criminal law standards that is a very low level of law-breaking. Prosecutions are even rarer.

Advocates of legalised assisted suicide suggest this means that the law is not working. For example, in 2009 Lord Falconer told the House of Lords that "*nobody wishes to prosecute in those cases, because nobody, in my view correctly, has the stomach to prosecute in cases of compassionate assistance*"[10]. In 2014 he stated that the courts and prosecuting authorities "*have tried to steer a course between Section 2 of the Suicide Act 1961 and the desire not to enforce it*"[11].

This view is open to question. The efficacy of a law is not to be judged by the number of prosecutions which result from it. The primary purpose of the criminal law is not to haul us through the courts or send us to prison but to deter unacceptable behaviour. Only when deterrence fails does the law's punitive role emerge. The small number of cases of assisting suicide and the low

---

[9] 6th Report 2015 (Session 4): Stage 1 Report on Assisted Suicide (Scotland) Bill, Paragraph 39

[10] House of Lords Hansard, 7 July 2009, Col. 596

[11] House of Lords Hansard, 18 July 2014 Col 775

prosecution rate are in reality two sides of the same coin. The serious penalties that the law holds in reserve are sufficient to make anyone minded to assist someone's suicide think very carefully indeed before proceeding. As a result the cases that do occur are few in number and tend to be those where assistance has been given reluctantly, after considerable thought and for genuinely compassionate reasons. These are cases that do not call for prosecution, and they are not prosecuted. They do not, however, provide a valid guide to the sort of cases which would occur under an advance licensing system.

Another argument sometimes heard is that the handful of cases of assisting suicide that cross the DPP's desk does not tell the whole story. The campaigning group Dignity in Dying (DiD) has suggested that *"terminally ill people are taking measures into their own hands by attempting to end their lives in unenviable circumstances"*[12]. This statement is based on responses from Directors of Public Health in England to a Freedom of Information Request by DiD in 2014. Only 6 out of 139 authorities identified terminal illness in their data on suicides. According to DiD, 7.36 per cent of this small sample of suicides involved people who had had a terminal illness. Applying this percentage to the total number of recorded suicides in 2012, DiD had calculated that some 332 suicides in that year had been of people who were terminally ill[13].

It is impossible, however, to know whether any of those who ended their lives would have met the other criteria for legalised assisted suicide which DiD believes should be part of an 'assisted dying' law - for example, whether they had had mental capacity or were free from external pressures or had had a settled wish to die. People take their own lives for many reasons and it is certainly

---

[12] 'The True Cost - How the UK outsources death to Dignitas', Dignity in Dying 2017

[13] A Hidden Problem: Suicide by Terminally Ill People, Dignity in Dying. October 2014

possible that a diagnosis of terminal illness could be a factor in some cases. There is research[14] indicating that the incidence of suicide attempts is higher in the period immediately following diagnosis but declines thereafter. There is also research[15] indicating that legalisation of assisted suicide does not reduce overall suicide rates. Whatever the position, it arguably points to a need for terminally ill people to receive better support - medical, psychological and social - rather than that they should be given help to take their own lives. However well-intentioned 'assisted dying' legislation may be, in effect it divides society into people whose suicides we should try to prevent and others (the terminally ill) whose suicides we should see it as appropriate to facilitate.

Is the law clear enough?

Advocates of legalisation recognise that the prosecution rate for assisting suicide is very low. However, they argue that someone who is contemplating giving assistance from wholly compassionate motives cannot be assured of immunity from prosecution and that, even in circumstances where a prosecution seems unlikely, a police investigation is nonetheless necessary and can prove a harrowing experience for someone who has just gone through the trauma of losing a loved one.

Any suspected case of assistance with suicide has to be investigated in order that a judgement can be reached of whether an offence has been committed and, if so, whether there has been criminality warranting prosecution. It is understandable that someone who from wholly compassionate motives has assisted a

---

[14] Bolton JM, Walld, R, Chateau D, Finlayson G, Sareen J 'Risk of suicide and suicide attempts associated with physical disorders: a population-based, balancing score-matched analysis', Psychological Medicine (2015) 45, 495-504

[15] Jones DA and Paton, D 'How does legalization of physician-assisted suicide affect rates of suicide', Southern Medical Journal, Volume 108, Number 10, October 2015

loved one to depart from this world may be concerned that there can be no assurance of non-prosecution until the case has been investigated and cleared.

Since 2010 it has been possible for someone who is contemplating assisting another person's suicide to know the kind of circumstances that will be taken into account by the DPP in reaching a decision. In that year, in response to a Judgment of what is now the Supreme Court, the Crown Prosecution Service published a document[16] setting out how decisions are made in such cases and listing various factors which might incline towards a decision to prosecute and others which might tend in the opposite direction. It states, for example, that a prosecution is more likely if there is evidence that the person whose suicide was assisted did not have mental capacity or had not expressed a voluntary and settled wish to die. Evidence that the assister had been motivated by the prospect of gain or had in some way applied pressure would tend in the same direction. On the other hand, a prosecution is less likely, says the policy, if there is evidence that the assister had been wholly motivated by compassion or had acted reluctantly or had given assistance which was relatively minor.

There are obvious dangers that such a published policy may be seen by some as giving them a green light to assist a suicide. The authors of the policy have therefore inserted some important caveats. They state:

> "*This policy does not in any way 'decriminalise' the offence of encouraging or assisting suicide. Nothing in this policy can be taken to amount to an assurance that a person will be immune from prosecution if he or she does an act that encourages or assists the suicide or the attempted suicide of another person*"[17]

---

[16] Policy for Prosecutors in Respect of Cases of Encouraging or Assisting Suicide, Crown Prosecution Service, 25 February 2010

[17] Ibid, Paragraph 6

They also warn against using the illustrative list of aggravating and mitigating factors as a simple checklist for deciding whether a prosecution will take place. Deciding whether or not a prosecution is in the public interest, says the policy, "*is not simply a matter of adding up the number of factors on each side and seeing which side has the greater number. Each case must be considered on its own facts and on its own merits...It is quite possible that one factor alone may outweigh a number of other factors which tend in the opposite direction*"[18].

In other words, the policy explains how the law is applied and how prosecuting decisions are made, and it provides an indication of the sort of circumstances which are taken into account in making such decisions. But it offers no guarantees. Every case has to be considered on its own merits.

The policy does not, however, satisfy those who want to see assisted suicide legalised. In their view not knowing in advance whether an act of assisted suicide will be prosecuted means that the law lacks clarity. And they suggest that it would not only reassure the assister but also help to protect the person whose suicide is assisted if the investigation were to take place before rather than after the death.

Prior immunity from prosecution cannot be given for any criminal act. If the Crown Prosecution Service were to do so, it would be acting in defiance of Parliament. The DPP has discretion to decide, in the light of all the evidence surrounding a specific offence, whether a prosecution is necessary in the public interest in that particular case. But to give an undertaking in advance of an act that it will not be prosecuted would be, in effect, to change the law. That is Parliament's prerogative.

It is fair to argue that uncovering criminal behaviour after the event comes too late for the person who has died. So would it not

---

[18] Ibid, Paragraph 39

be better to make sure there is no criminality before rather than after assistance with suicide is given? The trouble with this suggestion is that it does not compare like with like. A police investigation after the event is not infallible but it does focus on evidence and facts - on what has actually happened and in what circumstances. That is quite different from the pre-event assessment that advocates of legalisation have in mind. What they are proposing is a regime whereby assistance with suicide should be authorised on the basis of subjective opinions - about, for example, whether there is any coercion or other pressure at work in the background or about how settled is an apparent wish to end it all. We look more closely in Chapter Seven at just how reliable such assessments might be. Suffice it to say here that it is doubtful that they could be relied on to expose true intent or motivation in the same way as can an objective analysis of what has actually happened.

Nor should we underestimate the role of deterrence. Under the present law anyone minded to assist another person's suicide has to reckon with a spotlight being shone on his or her actions and on any criminal intent or behaviour coming to light as a result. Under a pre-event system of assessment, on the other hand, the only risk being run by someone with malicious intent is that the application might be rejected. Moreover, once assistance has been officially authorised, what is to prevent coercion or other pressure being applied between the time when the authorisation is given and the act of assistance itself? We should not forget that in those overseas jurisdictions which have legalised such practices there can often be a gap of weeks, months or sometimes even years between the two stages. In such cases exchanging post-event for pre-event scrutiny has the potential to put the person contemplating suicide at <u>increased</u> risk of malpractice.

But is it really assisting suicide?

It is commonly argued by advocates of legalised 'assisted dying' that what they are proposing is not assistance with suicide but assistance with dying. The essence of this argument is that, if we assist people who are not suffering from a terminal illness to end their lives, we are assisting a suicide; whereas, if we assist a terminally ill person out of this world, we are only assisting his or her dying - because we are hastening a death which is approaching from natural causes.

This distinction has no basis in law. If you end your own life deliberately, in law that is suicide; and a doctor or anyone else who knowingly supplies you with the means or otherwise helps you to do so is assisting suicide. Nonetheless the distinction between assisting the deaths of terminally and non-terminally ill people is one that will resonate with many people. Some might say that, if you know that you are going to die in the near future and you want to get it over with, that is surely not the same thing as wanting to end it all when you have your life in front of you.

No, it isn't the same thing. However, it is questionable whether this provides solid ground on which to build a case for legalisation. To say that it is permissible to help you to end your life if you have received a terminal prognosis but not if you haven't is to say that people who are terminally ill should be treated differently in law from people who are not. Some may perhaps see such differentiation as conferring a benefit on people who are terminally ill - in the form of desired assistance to end their lives. But it is necessary to see the other side of the coin. The law exists to protect us from harm - not just from others but also from ourselves - and it is arguable that a law which allows assistance with suicide for some but not for others is offering differing levels of protection to people in different health situations. On this interpretation an 'assisted dying' law could be said to run counter to one of the fundamental principles of legislation, that the law should protect all of us equally, irrespective of our age, gender, race - and state of health.

This is not to say, of course, that the law must never discriminate. Laws can be and have been made to give protection to specific groups of people who are considered to need it. However, when such laws are enacted, their purpose is usually to level the playing field and to ensure that everyone is treated equally. It is difficult to see an 'assisted dying' law in this light.

The distinction that is being drawn between 'assisted dying' and assisted suicide raises other questions. People who are incurably ill, for example with multiple sclerosis or Parkinson's disease, may not be dying in the sense that they are expected to die within a specified timeframe; but they are incurably ill and their conditions can be life-limiting. The difference between their medical state and that of others who have been declared to be terminally ill is essentially one of timeframe. This raises the question: if it is seen as an act of compassion to hasten the death of someone with a prognosis of a few months, why should similar action be viewed differently in the case of someone who will have to cope with an incurable condition for much longer?

Some advocates of legalisation have argued that there is a parallel between terminally ill people who end their lives prematurely and those people who, on 11 September 2001, jumped from the Twin Towers in New York to avoid being burned to death. The argument runs that, if those who jumped were not committing suicide (and few would say they were), then hastening an inevitable death from terminal illness cannot be seen as suicide.

This argument will not hold water. Those who jumped to their deaths on 9/11 were, like everyone else who died in that tragedy, the victims of external events. In jumping from the Twin Towers they were not choosing to die: they were choosing between two horrific forms of dying. A terminally ill person who swallows lethal drugs to hasten his or her death is not in the same position. The choice here is between dying of natural causes, supported by health care, and taking one's own life.

Suicidal intent is normally regarded as an indication of mental disturbance of one form or another. That is why doctors have a duty of care to take action to protect a patient who shows signs of suicidal thinking. The distinction that is drawn between a person who wants to kill himself because he does not want to go on living and someone else who wants to hasten an imminent death is not as straightforward as it might seem. Terminally ill people who want to hasten their deaths can sometimes be no-nonsense and strong-willed individuals who have been in control all their lives and want to remain in control to the end. But they can also be people who are seriously depressed (a frequent concomitant of terminal illness), who are struggling to come to terms with their mortality or are worried about the burden that their illness is placing on those around them. If they were not terminally ill, we would not consider for a moment helping them to take their own lives. So the question arises: why should we tell ourselves that because they are terminally ill we are not really assisting their suicide but simply assisting their dying?

The law and the courts

Recent years have seen a number of appeals, supported by campaigning groups for legalisation, seeking a Judgment from the courts that the existing law relating to assistance with suicide is in breach of human rights. At the time of writing these appeals have not resulted in any such Judgment. They raise, however, the constitutional question of the respective roles of Parliament and the courts in deciding whether the law should be changed.

It is for Parliament to legislate and thereby to decide what the law should be, while the role of the courts is to oversee the application of the law and, if necessary, to draw to the attention of Parliament any instance where it is considered that existing legislation may be in conflict with other laws or may be bearing with disproportionate severity on those affected. In the event that a senior court, whether the High Court, the Court of Appeal or the Supreme Court, should judge that to be so, it is for Parliament to consider whether in the light of that Judgement the law should be modified.

The respective roles of Parliament and the courts was the theme of Lord Jonathan Sumption's 2019 Reith Lecture. Lord Sumption had been a Justice of the Supreme Court from 2012 to 2018. In the course of his first lecture he addressed the issue of 'assisted dying' in response to a question from a member of the audience who argued that the existing law was 'broken' and was in need of change. Describing it as an issue *"on which people have strong moral views and on which they disagree"*, he posed the question: *"how do we resolve a disagreement like that?"* In his view, *"where there is a difference of opinion within a democratic community, we need a political process in order to resolve it"*. In other words, it is a matter for Parliament.

Asked by the BBC presenter, Anita Anand, to reveal his own view of whether the law should be changed Lord Sumption replied (it is worth quoting his reply in full) as follows:

> *"I'll tell you exactly what I think about this. I think that the law should continue to criminalise assisted suicide and I think that the law should be broken. I think that it should be broken from time to time. We need to have a law against it in order to prevent abuse but it has always been the case that this has been criminal and it has always been the case that courageous relatives and friends have helped people to die. And I think that is an untidy compromise of the sort that very few lawyers would adopt, but I don't believe that there is necessarily a moral obligation to obey the law. And ultimately it is something that each person has to decide within his own conscience"*[19].

[19] BBC Reith Lecture 2019, by kind permission of Profile Books

These words were direct and to the point, but their meaning is clear – that we need a law prohibiting assistance with suicide and that there will be rare occasions when that law might perhaps be broken for wholly-altruistic reasons. Elsewhere in his Reith Lecture Lord Sumption pointed to a need for *"a clear understanding of what the rule of law does not mean. It does not mean that every human problem and every moral dilemma calls for a legal solution"*.

So what conclusions can we draw?

There is a lot of talk about compassion in the 'assisted dying' debate. But the debate is not really about compassion. I have no problem accepting that in highly exceptional circumstances it could be the compassionate thing to do to accede to a request to help someone out of this life. The real question - and this takes us back to where we started - is whether the law should be changed to create a licensing system to facilitate such acts. That would represent a major change to the criminal law. It would be making it lawful to involve ourselves in deliberately bringing about the deaths of other people in certain circumstances. If Parliament is to be asked to take a decision of such gravity, it needs clear evidence, first, that the law that we have is not working; and, if that is the case, that what would be put in its place would be better.

In this chapter I have looked at the first of these questions - is the law as it stands fit for purpose? What we have seen is that the law is clear. We are left in no doubt what is unlawful, what the potential penalties are for breaking the law and how decisions are reached as to whether or not we will be prosecuted. Anyone contemplating assisting another's suicide can be in little doubt as to the likely consequences. Claims that the law is not clear do not stand up to serious examination.

In its report on whether assisted suicide should be legalised in Scotland, the Holyrood parliamentary committee (referred to above) noted :

> *"Although the uncertainty in the current law is perceived by some to be a disadvantage in the current position, this must be weighed against two advantages of the existing law: its ability to provide a strong deterrent as a safeguard against wrongdoing, and its ability to be sensitive to the facts of individual cases"*[20]

The law does not, and cannot, give immunity from prosecution. To do so would amount to changing the law. To suggest, as some do, that this absence of assurance means that the law lacks clarity is nonsense. As citizens, we have a right to know what the law is and how it is applied. We do not have a right to know in advance whether we will be prosecuted if we break the law in any individual case. Prosecution decisions must be fact-sensitive and must take account of the circumstances in which an offence has been committed, That cannot be done in advance.

A law may be clear but nonetheless oppressive. Is that the case here? It may be that the law prohibiting assistance with suicide is seen as oppressive by some individuals in specific circumstances. A scenario that is often rehearsed by advocates of legal change is that of a seriously ill person who goes to an assisted suicide facility in Switzerland while still able to travel in order to avoid implicating a family member who, at a later stage in the illness, might have to assist with the journey and thereby become liable to prosecution on returning to the UK.

The policy for prosecutors addresses situations such as this. It lists, as a potential mitigating factor in deciding whether a prosecution should take place, situations where the actions of the assister, "*although sufficient to come within the definition of the offence,*

[20] 6th Report 2015 (Session 4): Stage 1 Report on Assisted Suicide (Scotland) Bill, Paragraph 52

were of only minor encouragement or assistance". This does not give a blanket immunity from prosecution in such cases: every case is different and has to be examined on its own individual merits. But accompanying a family member, at his or her request, to the Dignitas assisted suicide facility in Zurich is perhaps the kind of 'minor assistance' that the policy has in mind.

Moreover, in considering whether the law is oppressive, we have to ask ourselves the question: oppressive for whom? The human-interest stories that are paraded before us in the media tend to be concerned with individuals who are strong-willed and determined to end their lives and who find the law's prohibition of assistance with suicide a nuisance. It is all too easy to forget that for most people, and especially for those who are seriously ill, life is less about asserting their will and more about coping with the circumstances of their lives, including pressures from others and from within themselves. It is to protect such people that the law exists. A law licensing assisted suicide may perhaps be seen as a blessing by a resolute and determined minority but it also has the potential to expose other, more vulnerable people to harm by increasing the pressures on them.

If the law is not oppressive, does it command social acceptance? This is an important test for any law to pass. If a law is widely flouted or resented, it cannot really be considered fit for purpose. We have seen that breaches of the law are rare - rarer than breaches of most other criminal laws. Even if we accept what the advocates of legalisation claim - that the few cases that cross the DPP's desk do not tell the whole story - the incidence of law-breaking in this area is nonetheless very small.

The law also reflects social attitudes to suicide. While it is widely agreed that people who attempt suicide should be treated with understanding and compassion, our society does not take the view that suicide is something to be encouraged or assisted. These social attitudes are reflected in the 'suicide watches' that are maintained where individuals are thought to be at risk of self-harm and in the suicide prevention strategies that successive governments have endorsed.

Advocates of legalisation point to opinion polling, which suggests that a substantial majority of people believe the law should be changed. I address the issue of opinion polling in more detail in Chapter Three. Suffice it to say here that public opinion and opinion polls are not necessarily the same thing and that what we say to opinion pollsters, on this as on a range of subjects, depends on the context of the questions put to us and on our understanding of the issues involved.

It is necessary also to beware of regarding the law as merely a regulatory instrument - as a means of bringing people to book if they have done something illegal. That is part of the purpose of legislation. But law-making has a wider aim than this. A fundamental aim of legislation is to state social values - to make clear which actions are regarded as unacceptable. Laws send social messages. If something is permitted by law, it carries with it a stamp of social approval. A law licensing doctors to supply lethal drugs to terminally ill people is more than just an escape road for a few individuals who want to end their lives. It also sends the message, however unintended, to others who are terminally ill that such practices have social approval and are worthy of consideration. As The Guardian wrote in 2014, on the day before a Private Member's Bill in the name of Lord Falconer was debated in the House of Lords, an 'assisted dying' law "*would create a new moral landscape*"[21].

---

[21] The Guardian 17 July 2014

CHAPTER TWO

THE DOCTOR'S DILEMMA

ILORA FINLAY

'Our duty of care...does not include being in any way part of their suicide'

We have talked so far about assisted suicide - because that is what the law is concerned with. But Parliament has been asked to consider - and has rejected - not just assisted suicide but *physician*-assisted suicide. What is being proposed is that doctors should be licensed by law to provide lethal drugs to terminally ill people who ask for them and are thought to meet certain criteria.

Those last seven words are very important. Under an 'assisted dying' law doctors would not just be licensed to provide terminally ill patients with the means to end their own lives. They would also be expected to decide who should and who should not qualify to receive such drugs[1]. We need to consider therefore the medical profession's view of this. Before doing so, however, it is necessary to look at how medical practice operates in the treatment of patients who are terminally ill.

---

[1] Though it has been suggested that doctors' decisions in such cases should be subject to endorsement by a judge of the High Court, that would not, as we will see in Chapter Seven, remove from them responsibility for making such decisions.

Medical Care at the End of Life

Choice and Control

Much of the debate on 'assisted dying' centres on the desire for choice and control at the end of life. In fact, we have more choice and control over our deaths than ever before, though its existence is not always appreciated. No doctor may lawfully treat us without our consent. There is no law against refusing treatment, including treatment that may save or extend our lives. A doctor may try to dissuade us from pursuing that course: doctors have - and, most people would agree, should have - a predisposition towards preserving life. But the decision whether to have life-saving or life-extending treatment is ours - and ours alone.

If we are worried that we might not be in a position to refuse treatment - for example, if a decision has to be made when we are unconscious - it is open to us to make a legally-binding Advance Decision to Refuse Treatment (ADRT). An ADRT enables us to specify situations in which we do not want to have certain medical treatments - for example, some people might not want to be resuscitated by chest compressions and defibrillation after a severe heart attack. In fact, only around 4 per cent of people in Britain make an ADRT.

So, if we can say to a doctor that we do not want treatment that will save or extend our lives, why can’t we ask a doctor to supply us with the means to bring our lives to an end? In reality the two situations are not comparable. A patient who refuses life-extending treatment is not, in doing so, expressing a wish to die but a willingness to let nature take its course. Neither in law nor in medical ethics does death as the result of treatment refusal constitute suicide. The difference between refusing live-prolonging treatment and requesting lethal drugs is the difference between accepting death and seeking death.

Patient choice is an essential feature of all medical care, but it does not mean that a patient may demand and receive any treatment or procedure that he or she wishes. It is more accurate to talk of patient consent than patient choice. Across medicine as a whole doctors may refuse to give treatments if they consider them to be harmful or unnecessary. In 2004 a retired professor of surgery, giving evidence to a House of Lords select committee[2], observed that "*the impression has been given that obeying patients' wishes is the overriding ethical imperative for doctors*". He told the committee:

> "*Of course it is important but it is not paramount. If it were, I would have done many unnecessary operations and some harmful operations in my time as a surgeon*"[3].

He reminded the committee that doctors sometimes refuse patients' demands for antibiotics for relatively trivial conditions because of the harmful downstream effects of over-prescribing on the community.

There already exists, therefore, a 'right to die'. What does not exist - but is often confused with a right to die - is a right to involve someone else in bringing about our deaths. It is also often not recognised that, if we opt to refuse life-extending treatment, our doctors still have a duty of care to ensure that we receive proper end-of-life care - ie medical care to relieve the pain or other symptoms of our illness as we die. It is not a choice between agreeing to treatment and being abandoned.

Open Discussion

Another claim often heard is that the law prevents dying people who want to bring their lives to an end from having an open and

---

[2] The committee is referred to hereinafter as the Mackay Committee from the name of its Chair, Lord Mackay of Clashfern

[3] House of Lords Report 86-I (Session 2004-05), Paragraph 45

frank dialogue on the subject with their doctors. There is nothing in law or in medical ethics to prevent patients discussing a wish to end their lives with their doctors. Indeed, given that doctors have an important role in suicide prevention, it is desirable that there should be a doctor-patient dialogue in such circumstances. A doctor cannot comply with a patient's request for assistance with suicide or take any action which might be construed as encouraging or assisting a patient to act in this way. But that does not preclude open and honest discussion of the patient's fears, feelings or wishes or exploration of how these might be resolved.

The position was explained with clarity by the General Medical Council in guidance issued to doctors in 2013. The relevant paragraph of the guidance states that:

> "*Where patients raise the issue of assisting suicide, or ask for information that might encourage or assist them in ending their lives, doctors should be prepared to listen and to discuss the reasons for the patient's request but they must not actively encourage or assist the patient as this would be a contravention of the law*".

The guidance goes on to say that "*doctors should continue to care for their patients and must be respectful and compassionate. We recognise that doctors will face challenges in ensuring that patients will not feel abandoned while ensuring that the advice or encouragement that they provide does not encourage or assist suicide. Doctors are not required to provide treatments that they consider will not be of overall benefit to the patient or which will harm the patient. Respect for a patient's autonomy cannot justify illegal action*"[4].

---

[4] Guidance for Investigation Committee and case examiners when considering allegations about a doctor's involvement in encouraging or assisting suicide, GMC January 2013

These are by their nature sensitive areas of discussion, and difficulties may conceivably arise in some cases - for example, if a patient does not seek direct assistance with suicide but requests, say, a letter of referral with the intention of seeking such assistance abroad where it is legal. But the message is clear - if a patient talks of a wish to 'end it all', the doctor should engage in discussion in order to explore what is going on in the patient's thinking and to see whether and how the situation can be resolved or alleviated. An important part of medical training today is to ensure that doctors understand the importance of listening to their patients respectfully and with an open mind.

Doctor-Patient Trust

If patient consent is a cardinal feature of clinical practice, even more fundamental is trust between patient and doctor. We need to be able to take it for granted that our doctors will always act in our best interests and, at the least, that the treatment or advice we receive from them will (in the words of the Hippocratic Oath) 'do no harm'. Can this trust be maintained in a situation where we are asking doctors to involve themselves in deliberately bringing about our deaths? Does legalising physician-assisted suicide pose risks to doctor-patient trust?

Advocates of legalisation argue that, where 'assisted dying' in one form or another has been legalised, patients say they continue to trust their doctors. Of course they do, but the argument misses the point. We trust our doctors, not because the law says this or that, but because we need medical care and they have been judged qualified to provide it. In much the same way we trust the pilots of the airliners we board, not because we are content with the rules governing flight safety, but because we need to travel by air and they have been judged qualified to fly us. The emergence of an occasional rogue professional does not seem to undermine this trust, which is to a large extent born of necessity.

However, I would suggest that the question has been posed the wrong way round. It is not so much whether patients continue to trust their doctors under a regime of physician-assisted suicide that is at issue here, but whether the existence of that trust makes them more vulnerable under such a regime. The doctor-patient relationship is, for most of us, a highly asymmetric one, in which the doctor holds most of the cards. The doctor has professional knowledge and experience which most patients are not in a position to challenge. There can also be an emotional asymmetry - for example, in situations where seriously ill patients are anxious and look to their doctors for guidance and reassurance. The doctor-patient relationship is not just another customer-supplier relationship. It is one in which the doctor has a duty of care and a responsibility to act in the patient's best interests. It is easy to scoff at this, as some do, as medical paternalism. But it lies at the heart of clinical practice. A good doctor is more than just a diagnostician or prescriber. He (or she) sees the patient as a whole: fears, wishes, beliefs and values as well as symptoms and scans. The doctor guides as well as treats.

So, what happens when we introduce into this complex relationship the concept of physician-assisted suicide? Seriously ill patients can and sometimes do talk to their doctors about wanting help to end it all. Some (a tiny number in the experience of most doctors) may really want to end their lives. But it is another, much larger group who are of most concern in this context - patients who talk about 'giving me something to end it all', not because they have come to a clear decision to end their lives but as a means of signalling that they are up against it and as a way of opening up the topic of their own dying in order to establish more clearly whether their fears, whatever they may be, are warranted and what lies ahead of them. In cases such as these doctor-patient trust comes seriously into play. A good doctor will listen carefully to the patient to find out what lies behind the request - is it the treatment regime? or something that is going on at home? Is the patient fearful of something that is extremely unlikely to happen or suffering from depression? In a word, what can be done to alleviate the situation?

Now consider the same scenario where a physician-assisted suicide regime is in place. The doctor may well handle the request in the same way, talking matters through with the patient and providing assurance and an improved treatment regime. It depends very much on who the doctor is: like their patients, doctors are not a homogeneous group. However, a doctor who interprets such a request as a wish to die and agrees to explore physician-assisted suicide risks sending the message to the patient, albeit unintentionally, that in his or her circumstances a hastened death might well be, in the doctor's professional opinion, the best course of action - at least an option worth considering. For strong-willed patients who are clear in their minds that they want to end their lives, and around whom the campaigning for legalisation is largely focused, this may make little difference. But they are few and are considerably outnumbered by other, more vulnerable patients who are deeply reliant on the doctor-patient relationship and who, not unreasonably, could easily interpret a doctor's willingness to process a request for lethal drugs as meaning that, in the doctor's view, what lies ahead is so awful that taking their own lives is a medically sensible option.

In reality, therefore, it is the very existence of doctor-patient trust and the inherent asymmetry of the doctor-patient relationship that makes legalising physician-assisted suicide potentially dangerous. The Royal College of Physicians recognised this in a letter which it wrote to the Director of Public Prosecutions in December 2009. The College wrote that "*the trust afforded doctors and nurses in particular gives their views considerable weight with their patients and the public*" and warned that the involvement of doctors in assisting suicide was "*open to misinterpretation*"[5]. The

[5] Letter from Royal College of Physicians to Director of Public Prosecutions dated 14 December 2009

final version of the policy for prosecutors, when it was published in February 2010, included, as a potentially aggravating factor in an act of assisting suicide, a situation where the assister "*was acting in his or her capacity as a medical doctor, nurse, other healthcare professional, a professional carer, or as a person in authority, such as a prison officer, and the victim was in his or her care*"[6].

This section of the policy for prosecutors has been a source of controversy on both sides of the 'assisted dying' debate. Advocates of legalisation have argued that it encourages 'amateur' assistance with suicide. This argument is difficult to sustain. The policy does not encourage any kind of assistance with suicide. It does not say that assistance with suicide must not be provided by a qualified doctor but that a doctor's assistance in the suicide of a patient who was in his or her care could be seen as a breach of doctor-patient trust. However, in June 2014 the Supreme Court, in response to an appeal, invited the DPP to consider whether the meaning of the policy in this respect should be clarified. The DPP responded, in October 2014, by underlining the words "*the victim was in his or her care*".

This clarification was, in turn, challenged by opponents of legalisation. The reasoning behind the challenge appeared to be that, in emphasising that medical assistance with suicide would be regarded as aggravated where a previous duty of care had existed, there was an implication that medical assistance with suicide was not regarded as an aggravation in other circumstances. On this interpretation, it could perhaps be argued that the underlining might be seen as encouraging a small number of doctors who may be ideologically committed to the principle of 'assisted dying' to engage in assisting the suicides of people with whom they had had no previous professional relationship.

---

[6] Policy for Prosecutors in Respect of Cases of Encouraging or Assisting Suicide, CPS 25 February 2010, Paragraph 43

However, the words could be said to have been open to that misinterpretation before the DPP's clarification; the underlining did no more than make clear what the policy was intended to mean. Unsurprisingly, in December 2015 the High Court rejected the challenge.

Covert Euthanasia

Are doctors in Britain acting outside the law and covertly ending patients' lives? Are end-of-life decisions exposed to proper scrutiny? Professor Clive Seale, who has conducted extensive research in this area, told Lord Falconer's Commission on Assisted Dying that his surveys of end-of-life decision-making by UK doctors had found no reports of physician-assisted suicide and half a percent of deaths as the result of euthanasia and that these figures were lower than in other countries where the same surveys had been done.

Commenting on his findings, Professor Seale said:

> *"In the UK doctors are particularly collegiate; they like to share their decisions, not just with patients and relatives, but also with each other and with nursing staff as well. There is a kind of joint quality to decision-making in the UK medical practice that is very marked compared to other countries. And with that situation decisions don't go unscrutinised"*[7].

As to illegal activity by doctors, Professor Seale felt that *"it does sometimes happen in UK medical practice but pretty rarely"*. Research into end-of-life decision-making by UK doctors published in 2009 concluded that in the UK *"euthanasia, physician assisted suicide and the ending of life without an explicit patient request ('involuntary euthanasia') are rare or non-existent"*[8].

---

[7] Commission on Assisted Dying, Oral Evidence 14 December 2010

[8] Seale, C. End of Life Decisions in the UK involving medical practitioners, Palliative Medicine 2009; 00:1-7

Nonetheless the notion that doctors may be hastening the deaths of seriously-ill patients surfaces from time to time and it is important to ask why this should be. Distressed relatives may misinterpret the administration of analgesics or other symptom-relieving drugs to their dying loved ones as covert euthanasia. They see injections being given and their loved ones dying afterwards, and they may mistakenly link the two as cause and effect. In the emotional turmoil of losing a relative such misinterpretation can become magnified. In a person who is close to death from an underlying illness there will always be a last injection of medication, just as there will always be a last visit from a family member or a last cup of tea.

Increased dosages of analgesia can occasionally be needed to provide more effective pain relief in patients whose care has become very complex through a wide range of interacting factors that have made relief of distress more difficult. It is possible that this could in very rare circumstances lead to respiration being depressed and to an inadvertent hastening of a patient's death. In such a situation, where hastening of death is an unintended side-effect of pain relief, a doctor would be acting within the bounds of the law and of medical ethics. This is the principle known as 'double effect'. It can be seen in other branches of medicine – for example, in surgery, where operations may be performed for a patient's benefit but may not be entirely without risk.

In modern end-of-life care 'double effect' situations are extremely rare. Pain-relief is a sophisticated science these days and it is possible to administer effective symptom relief without hastening the death of the patient. In fact, the reverse can often be the case. There has been evidence that patients receiving good symptom control, with pain controlled with adequate doses of morphine and other medication, live longer on average and with higher quality of life scores than those who do not receive expert palliative care input for optimal symptom control [9] [10].

In modern UK clinical practice, where care of the dying is a specialised branch of medicine, where pharmacists monitor prescriptions and medication stocks, and where teamwork encourages transparency of behaviour, covert euthanasia would be very difficult to practice with impunity. This is not to say that deliberate ending of life never happens: human nature being what it is, it is impossible to rule out malpractice completely. But the notion that doctors deliberately end the lives or hasten the deaths of patients as part of good compassionate care does not rest on any serious evidence.

How Doctors See 'Assisted Dying'

It is time now to return to the question posed at the beginning of this chapter: what view does the medical profession take of legalisation? There are two aspects to this question - how doctors themselves view 'assisted dying' and what view the medical professional bodies take.

Surveys of opinion among doctors suggest that the majority do not support a change in the law. A Medeconnect poll of 1,000 GPs in May 2015[11] indicated that just 14 per cent (one in seven) would be willing to conduct a full assessment of a request for assisted suicide, though 39 per cent said that they might be willing to give a professional opinion on strictly-medical aspects of a request to another decision-maker, such as a court. Among doctors who specialise in treatment and care of the dying opposition to 'assisted dying' is even higher, with more than nine out of ten doctors expressing unwillingness to participate.

---

[9] Temel JS et al NEJM 2010;363:733-42

[10] Higginson et al Lancet Respiratory Medicine, Dec 2014; 2(12): 979-987

[11] Medeconnect Poll of GPs May 2015

Advocates of legalisation argue that the medical profession should stand back and not oppose what, according to opinion polls, a majority of the public say they want. It is, they suggest, a matter for society as a whole rather than for the medical profession. In a letter to The Times in April 2015, after that paper had urged caution in regard to legalisation and had drawn attention to doctors' concerns, the late Lord Joffe, a leading supporter of legalisation, wrote to express surprise *"that The Times is of the view that the opposition of a majority of doctors should prevail over the views of the 82 per cent of society who support the legalisation of assisted dying. It is for society through the parliamentary process to determine our laws*[12].

Lord Joffe was right to point out that it is for Parliament to decide whether the law should be changed. But no one is suggesting that the opposition of the majority of doctors should be the deciding factor in whether 'assisted dying' should be legalised. Parliament is at liberty to ignore the views of doctors if it thinks that is appropriate. It should not, however, be prevented from hearing those views and attaching appropriate weight to them. After all, doctors would be in the front line of implementing any assisted suicide law and they have first-hand experience of the vulnerabilities of seriously ill patients. Advocates of legalisation have argued that no group within society should have disproportionate influence in the debate. Disproportionate, no; but the influence of any person or group must surely be commensurate with their knowledge or experience of the subject and potential involvement in what is proposed.

It is also arguably inconsistent to appeal to public opinion polls in favour of legalising assisted suicide but to disregard surveys of medical opinion against legalising *physician*-assisted suicide. If it is insisted that these practices should be embedded within medicine, it is not unreasonable to listen to those whom we are asking to

---

[12] The Times, Letters 5 April 2015

perform them. The adage 'no decision about me without me' is one that is surely applicable here.

So what position have the medical professional bodies adopted? The BMA and Royal College of General Practitioners have expressed their opposition to legalisation. In 2010, when the DPP was conducting a public consultation prior to finalising his policy for prosecutors, the Royal College of Physicians (RCP) wrote to him that "*we believe that our duty of care is to work with patients to mitigate and overcome their clinical difficulties and suffering. It is clear to us that this does not include being, in any way, part of their suicide*"[13]. The College's opposition to a change in the law was re-affirmed following a survey of its fellows and members in 2014. However, in March 2019 the College announced, following another consultation, that it would be adopting a position of neutrality over whether the law should be changed.

In the 2019 consultation respondents were asked whether the RCP should support, oppose or be neutral on legalisation of 'assisted dying'. 31.6 per cent voted for the College to support a change in the law, 43.4 per cent voted that the College should remain opposed to legalisation and 25 per cent thought the RCP should be neutral. So the College adopted the position advocated by the least number of respondents - neutrality.

In announcing the change the College explained that neutrality "*reflects the lack of a simple majority for any particular view*"[14]. Whether or not there is a majority for any stance depends crucially on how the term 'majority' is defined. A majority vote is normally regarded as a vote that is greater in size than other votes. On this definition there was indeed a clear majority view - that the RCP should maintain its stance of opposition. There was not an *overall*

---

[13] Letter from Royal College of Physicians to Director of Public prosecutions dated 14 December 2009

[14] 'No majority view on assisted dying moves RCP position to neutral', RCP Press Release 21 March 2019

majority - ie a vote which was greater in size than the votes for all other views combined. But that was also the position in 2014, when the RCP reaffirmed its opposition to a change in the law.

Some supporters of legalised 'assisted dying' have argued that the recent consultation indicates that a majority of respondents (the 56.6 per cent who voted for Support or Neutrality) were not opposed to a change in the law. But the converse of this is also true. If the Oppose and Neutral vote shares are combined, an even larger majority (68.4 per cent) could be said to be not supportive of a change in the law.

There are two situations in which a consultation might justifiably be regarded as having pointed to a stance of neutrality. One is where respondents were asked to choose between two positions (support for or opposition to 'assisted dying') and the votes for each were evenly balanced. The other is where respondents were offered three options (support for, opposition to or neutrality on 'assisted dying') and neutrality received the largest number of votes. Neither of these situations applied in the recent consultation and the College has ended up with a position which the smallest number (just one in four) of its fellows and members supported.

It is worth looking at the breakdown of opinion by clinical specialty of those who responded to the consultation. Only 5 per cent of palliative medicine specialists expressed support for 'assisted dying', as did just 23 per cent of those engaged in geriatric medicine. Both are specialties much of whose work involves care of the elderly and/or terminally ill. By contrast, among those expressing support for 'assisted dying' were respondents from specialities with little or no day-to-day clinical responsibility for care of the dying, including tropical medicine, obstetrics and medical students.

In March 2020 the RCP published a statement making its position clear:

"Neutrality was defined as neither supporting nor opposing a change in the law, to try to represent the breadth of views within its membership. Regrettably, this position has been interpreted by some as suggesting that the College is either indifferent to legal change or is supportive of a change in the law.

"So that there can be no doubt, the RCP clarifies that it does not support a change in the law to permit assisted dying at the present time[15]".

Conclusion

The advocates of legalisation are right when they say that this is a matter for society as a whole. Many, if not most, of the factors in any desire for assistance with suicide are personal or social rather than medical. Assessing these is about balancing the wishes of individuals against the interests of the wider community. This is not something that doctors are trained or experienced to do. Their role is to treat illness where they can and to mitigate its symptoms where they cannot. Given the asymmetric nature of the doctor-patient relationship they must, of necessity, act in what they consider to be the best interests of their patients, even if this sometimes conflicts with what patients say they want. The doctor-patient relationship is not just another customer-supplier relationship. If patients are to be able to place themselves in doctors' hands with confidence, they need to know that, in advising or in treating them, their doctors will proceed from the 'do no harm' principle and from a presumption in favour of preserving lives.

To say this is not to argue for life at any cost. Most doctors can recognise when death has to be accepted and when over-zealous interventions are inappropriate. Clinicians of all disciplines are now better trained in the core principles of palliative and end-of-life care, can recognise when death is approaching and can talk

---

[15] RCP Press Release 26 March 2020

openly with their patients and the patient’s family about what is happening. As all come to accept the inevitability of death, they must continue to monitor all aspects of comfort to ensure that death is gentle and peaceful.

It is also permissible, both in law and in medical ethics, for a doctor to increase dosages of medication in exceptional cases in order to relieve pain or other distress even if there is a slight risk that doing so might unintentionally hasten the patient's death. With modern techniques of analgesia such situations are extremely rare these days and, where they do occur, their intention is to kill the pain, not the patient. These situations are, however, radically different from acting with the deliberate intention of bringing about a patient's death. That is the Rubicon which would be crossed if doctors were to be licensed to supply lethal drugs to some of their patients. It is not difficult to see, therefore, why the majority of them are opposed to such a change in the law.

Chapter Three

A Matter for Society

Robert Preston

We have as a society become less familiar with death and dying and less inclined to see these events as a natural and inevitable part of life

There is a paradox at the heart of the 'assisted dying' debate. Fifty or sixty years ago, when palliative medicine was in its infancy, it was not uncommon for people to die in severe pain or other distress. Yet there was no political pressure for legalising 'assisted dying'. Today pain-relief is a sophisticated science and palliative medicine has made huge advances in relieving the distress of incurable illness. There are still painful or otherwise distressing deaths, but they are considerably fewer than was once the case. Yet in parallel with these advances in medical science we are seeing political lobbying to change to law to license 'assisted dying'. How can this paradox be explained?

It is not only medicine that has changed over the last half century. Our perceptions of death and dying have changed too. In this chapter I want to touch on a few of these changes and to see how they influence the end-of-life debate.

Life Expectancy

It is undeniable that most of us are living longer. My grandfather died in the 1940s when he was 67, my grandmother in the early 1950s when she was 74. In both cases it was felt that they had had what used to be called 'a good innings'. My parents died some 40 years later in their eighties. Today anyone who dies at the traditional three-score-years-and-ten might be inclined to feel short-changed.

As a society we have come to expect to live to a ripe old age. Indeed, it is the increasing reality of these expectations that is beginning to raise difficulties over the affordability of health care and pensions. When the first British state pension was introduced in 1909, it was available to those aged 70 and over. Yet average life expectancy at the time was 48 for men and 55 for women. Today we expect to draw our pensions in our sixties and to go on living for a further 20 or more years.

However, the consequences go well beyond pensions. Living longer has changed the way we see death and dying. Earlier generations were more aware of death than we are - because they saw more of it. Some years ago I embarked on family history research and I was surprised, when I examined records of births, marriages and deaths in the mid-nineteenth century for the part of the country where I was brought up, to see how many children died then in childhood and how few adults survived until the age of 60. By the time I arrived on the scene 100 years later the situation was rather different. But death was still a more common feature of everyday life in the 1950s than it is today.

When something happens regularly, we accustom ourselves to it and we manage it. Today death is a less frequent visitor and, as with other things that are unfamiliar, it can inspire fear and terror. The situation was summed up well in a paper written a few years ago by Dr Charles Skinner, a palliative medicine consultant:

> "*We have as a society become less familiar with death and dying and less inclined to see these events as a natural and inevitable part of life. Within the memory of many people alive today death and dying were once everyday occurrences and there was a*

general recognition that potentially fatal illness could arise at any time.

"This contrasts markedly with attitudes to death today. We take good health and a long life for granted. It is possible to reach well into one's adult years without ever experiencing a bereavement of a close relative or friend. Death and debility have increasingly been banished to hospitals, hospices or nursing homes, with doctors and nurses taking over much of the responsibility for day-to-day care as well as clinical treatment.

"This shift in our experience of the dying process has meant that what was once commonplace and integrated into our daily lives has become remote and unfamiliar. As a result the prospect of witnessing the typical phases of someone's death can be daunting, in a way it was not to earlier generations, and the thought of having to experience the process of dying oneself can be a terrifying prospect to some. It is not surprising therefore that the response to diagnoses of life-limiting illness can sometimes be anger or indignation"[1].

In her book 'With the End in Mind'[2] another consultant in palliative medicine, Dr Kathryn Mannix, writes that "*death has become increasingly taboo*". She writes:

"Not knowing what to expect people take their cues instead from vicarious experience: television, films, novels, social media and the news. These sensational yet simultaneously trivialised versions of dying and death have replaced what was once everyone's common experience of observing the dying of people around them, of seeing death often enough to recognise its patterns, to become familiar with life lived well within the limits of decreasing vigour and even to develop a familiarity with the sequences of the deathbed".

---

[1] 'Palliative Care: What is it? And what has it got to do with 'assisted dying'? Published by Living and Dying Well

[2] 'With the End in Mind', Kathryn Mannix, published by William Collins 2017

"*That rich wisdom*", she writes, "*was lost in the second half of the twentieth century*". Advances in medical science and new life-prolonging treatments "*triggered a behaviour change that saw the sickest people being rushed into hospital for treatment instead of waiting at home to die*".

The wish to keep death at arm's length continues even after the event. At one time the bodies of people who had died were brought home, and relatives and friends came to pay their respects and take their farewells before the funeral. Today, except in a few parts of the United Kingdom, when we die we await burial or cremation at the funeral director's premises. Children are often now kept away from funerals, which are thought to be depressing for them. We no longer see death as a natural ending to life but rather as something to be put out of our thoughts for as long as we can, to be deplored when it approaches and to be managed by professionals when it occurs. Death, one might almost say, has become detached from life.

There is, however, another aspect of living longer that is also changing our attitudes to death. Many of us may be living longer lives but we are not always living longer and healthy lives. Before the days of penicillin, immunisation and vaccination we could be carried off by illnesses like pneumonia, diphtheria or smallpox - there were still occasional epidemics of these and other infectious diseases as recently as the 1960s. They were distressing illnesses but, when they were fatal, they tended to do their work quickly. As we have begun to live longer, we have become more susceptible to longer-lasting and degenerative conditions, often though not invariably associated with ageing, such as multiple sclerosis, Parkinson's disease, heart disease and dementia.

It is cause for celebration that advances in medical science have enabled us to extend our lives. For many people, living longer can bring a new lease of life. But that is not the case for everyone and it would not be surprising if, as times passes, we begin to see increasing numbers of people who genuinely do not want to go on living - who are just tired of life. The problem of longevity is one which as a society we are going to have to address.

Attitudes to Health Care

Health stories are rarely out of the news these days. If it is not a scare like Bird Flu in Asia, Ebola in Africa, Zika virus in South America or Coronavirus around the world, it is alleged shortcomings of the NHS. Health stories make good copy, partly because they are about something which affects us all and to which we can easily relate and partly because the condition of public healthcare services is a recognised political football. However, stories about health care, like other subjects of media attention, can convey a distorted picture.

Our attitudes to health care have changed markedly since the NHS was established. In the early days there was a recognition that, though medicine was advancing, there were limits to what it could do. A fair proportion of patients in those days were of a generation that was accustomed to seeking medical treatment only when strictly necessary. Seventy years on, the range of treatments, along with the cost, has increased dramatically and at the same time we have come to see health care as a citizen's right. We are told time and again that, if we should have this or that symptom, we should consult our doctors. It is little wonder that the system gets overloaded.

There is, however, another paradox here. Earlier generations were familiar with the colloquial phrase 'doctor's orders' - meaning what a doctor had advised us to do, or (more often) refrain from doing, in order to avoid illness or to speed recovery from an ailment. Yet alongside this apparent paternalism there was an acceptance that doctors, like anyone else, could make mistakes. Today we see this situation turned on its head. 'Doctor's orders' have gone and the emphasis is on patient choice. Yet, though we insist we are the ones in control, we find it difficult to forgive when doctors get it wrong – as, being human, they sometimes do.

The 'Baby Boomers'

It is not just a matter of living longer. There are other factors at work. My generation is that of the so-called baby-boomers. We are the generation born immediately after the Second World War and it has to be said that we have had it easier than other generations both before and since. After the horrendous sacrifices of two world wars there was, in the immediate post-war decades, a sense of 'never again' in the air and a determination to give the rising generation opportunities that their parents and grandparents had never had. We can see this dynamic at work in the passing of the 1944 Education Act, in the foundation in 1948 of the National Health Service and, from the 1950s onwards, in the promotion of full employment and the consumer society. As Prime Minister Harold Macmillan put it in the late 1950s, many people alive had 'never had it so good'.

I know what he meant. I received a first-rate (and free) grammar school education; a government grant to go to university, with tuition fees paid; a virtually-guaranteed entry into the professions on graduation; and the promise of a final-salary, index-linked pension on retirement. As my son put it to me when he started work in the 1990s in rather less favourable conditions, I had been in the right place and at the right time for just about everything on offer.

Nor was it just those of us who had gone into higher education who benefited. For the 20 years or so that followed the end of the war there was near-full employment; and everyone who bought his or her first home in the 50s, 60s and 70s had an opportunity to amass substantial capital assets for later in life. It is little wonder that we have been called the lucky generation.

However, this generation is now entering old age and coming face to face with something - death and dying - that cannot simply be air-brushed out of our lives or accommodated to our wishes. We have grown accustomed to living in peace, prosperity and security, to having our ailments treated, to expectations of a long life and to having our own way generally. It was not like this for earlier generations, who had to live with the threats of unemployment, poverty, war and fatal illnesses hanging over them. To them death was just one unpredictable event among many to have to cope with. To us, on the other hand, it comes in stark contrast to everything we have experienced. Having been placed in control of our lives in a way no previous generation in history has been, we have come up against something that we cannot control. And we don't like it.

Prosperity

Our society as a whole has attained a level of material prosperity which would have been beyond belief not only 100 but even 50 years ago. It has to be said that it is a very uneven prosperity - between north and south, between young and old and between different kinds of commodity. And there have been legitimate concerns expressed of a growing devil-take-the-hindmost approach to living. For that reason the words 'as a whole' are an important qualification. But from a strictly material point of view most people in Britain today live more comfortable and more prosperous lives than was ever the case in human history.

This rise in prosperity is something to be celebrated: it is a considerable achievement. But it has a downside. Prosperity opens up opportunities to assert ourselves, which is conducive to the growth of individualism and to a decline in social cohesion. A society is most cohesive when its members are inter-dependent. When we feel we are able to look after ourselves, we depend less on others and, conversely, we are less inclined to have them dependent on us. This rise in individualism has been one of the most marked features of the last few decades.

We are prosperous in more than just material possessions. We live in a society which prides itself on the provision of free health care, benefits, social services and pensions. Again, these provisions do not always match individual needs and there are many who are or feel excluded. But the situation is very different from that of previous generations, especially those who lived before the advent of the welfare state, who had to pay for or go without medical treatment, who could not rely on pensions to support them in their old age and who were in dire straits if they found themselves out of work. All in all, life for most people today is not only materially prosperous but comfortable too. And, when we are comfortably-placed, we are less willing to move on and inclined to be resentful when faced with the prospect.

Family Life

The last 50 years have also witnessed significant changes in family relationships. The opening up of higher education after the war made this inevitable. Whereas at one time a son or daughter would normally settle in the same area as the rest of the family, graduate employment usually involved going to where the job was, which often meant far from the rest of the family. I am a typical example of this phenomenon, having been brought up in Lancashire but obliged to spend my working life in the London area. One result of this was that my children, when they were young, met their grandparents no more than perhaps twice a year. The decline of the extended family began before the war but in the years after 1945 it accelerated.

The late 1960s saw divorce law reform. We now have many one-parent families and people living alone and often away from their children. The single-parent family is now a significant element in society.

As a result of these changes there is less integration between the generations than was once the case. When elderly people become ill or infirm, many do not have children or other family members nearby to whom they can turn for support. Even when they do, provision of support is often not straightforward. With soaring house prices and large mortgages to service many families need two incomes to keep their heads above water and they are in no position for one of their wage-earners to give up work to care for an ailing relative. There is consequently a growing problem of isolation among the elderly. The stronger among them are - or, of necessity, become - independent-minded. The less robust can face a life of loneliness and develop an inward-looking mentality, which in turn can have the effect of isolating them still further from the community around them.

The Choice Agenda

Choice has become a dominant force in politics and society today. In the decades immediately following the end of the war there was little choice in people's lives. Much of life was governed by monolithic organisations dealing with such things as transport, telephones, utilities and broadcasting. This was the era of post-war corporatism, which began to collapse with the economic management revolution of the 1980s. A similar process happened at around the same time in international relations, when the Berlin Wall fell and power blocks began to dissolve into individual States. In both cases a major contributing factor was the advent of new technologies which both thrived in and promoted individualistic rather than corporate societies.

An important consequence of this has been the growth of the choice agenda. We are now invited to mix and match all kinds of things in our lives, from broadcasting to mobile phone and internet 'packages', utilities, fare structures, schools and hospitals. For those who are able to handle it, it is an agreeable lifestyle and I would not wish to go back to the old one-size-fits-all days. But it is not without its problems. Choice is a great thing to have if you know what you want and you understand how to get it. But not everyone is in that happy position. A few years ago I had to have minor surgery and I was slightly taken aback when my GP asked me at which hospital I would like to have the operation. Having no knowledge as to the relative merits of the hospitals in the area I could only reply: 'A Good One'?

The same technologies that have promoted choice have fostered something else too. Many of the new technologies that we have in our lives today are such as to encourage us to operate as individuals rather than as members of a community. Concerns are sometimes expressed that children come home from school and engage with computer screens and smart phones rather than with other children. How often do we see people walking down the street or sitting on buses and trains who are plugged into music or other devices or scanning mobile-phone screens and, it can seem, are oblivious of those around them. The mobile phone is itself an assertion of individuality: it is not the house phone or the office phone, but a personal phone.

Some suggest that the internet and social media are a counter-current in this drift to individualism. I am doubtful of this. As many of us have discovered during the 2020 Coronavirus 'lockdown', an important part of community life is face-to-face contact, involving not just words and pictures but body language.

I would not wish to be misunderstood. This is not a Hovis-style commercial. I am not suggesting that life was better in the 1950s than it is now or that we should put the clock back. Social change is inevitable and it is to be welcomed, embraced and put to good use. But it is salutary to stand still from time to time and to look back and see how and why we have changed. To do so gives us a better chance of managing the future successfully. I have drawn attention to just a few of the changes that have taken place because they help to explain why, if we believe opinion polling, there is substantial public support for a change in the law. So let us turn now to the opinion polls.

Public Opinion

We need to start by recognising that public opinion and opinion polls are not the same thing. Opinion polls can give us a snapshot of what a small cross-section of the public says about this or that issue at a particular time and in response to a specific question or questions. But they can be misleading as a guide to what people really think. What people tell the pollsters depends on a number of factors - in particular, what question is asked? what is the context - for example, have there been recent press stories on the subject and how have they been presented? and what familiarity do the respondents have with the matter in question?

The Questions Asked

Let us look at a typical public opinion poll on the subject of 'assisted dying'. During March 2019 5,700 people were asked this question in an online poll[3]:

> *"Currently it is illegal for a doctor to help someone with a terminal illness to end their life, even if the person considers their suffering unbearable and they are of sound mind. A proposed new law would allow terminally ill adults the option of assisted dying. This would mean being provided with life-ending medication, to take themselves, if two doctors were satisfied they met all of the safeguards. They would need to be of sound mind, be terminally ill and have 6 months or less to live, and a High Court judge would have to be satisfied that they had made a voluntary, clear and settled decision to end their life, with time to consider all other options. Whether or not you would want the choice for yourself, do you support or oppose this proposal for assisted dying becoming law?"*

---

[3] Populus, Dignity in Dying Survey, Fieldwork 11-24 March 2019

Some of the words or phrases used in this question - 'for a doctor to help'; 'unbearable suffering'; 'option'; 'medication'; 'all the safeguards'; 'a High Court judge'; 'voluntary, clear and settled decision'; 'choice' – have the potential to reassure the sceptical respondent. But they can be misunderstood.

For example, the reference to doctors and terminal illness is irrelevant: the law prohibits assistance with suicide being given <u>by</u> anyone (not just doctors) and <u>to</u> anyone (not just people who have a terminal illness). Mention of doctors and illness, however, can be misconstrued as suggesting there might be a tension between the existing law and medical treatment. Lethal drugs are referred to as 'medication' - a contradiction and one that masks the reality of what is meant. The person being polled is not told what the 'safeguards' are. In reality, as we will see in Chapter Seven, all that is being offered by campaigning groups as regards safeguards is a few broadly-worded criteria.

Against this background it is hardly surprising if a substantial majority of people say they support a change in the law. The poll is effectively asking people whether they support the concept of 'assisted dying', to which many people can assent if it is expressed in those terms. Anyone who watched the *Yes, Prime Minister* television series in the 1980s will remember the episode in which Permanent Secretary Sir Humphrey Appleby demonstrates to the hapless Bernard Woolley how the results of opinion polling can be influenced by the language in which questions are asked.

In fact, the Mackay Committee, as part of its parliamentary inquiry into 'assisted dying', invited the public to write or email with their views. The results are revealing. Of more than 12,000 responses received before the closing date, 50.6 per cent supported a change in the law while 49.4 per cent opposed it[4]. If people take the trouble to write letters or emails to parliamentarians, it may be

[4] House of Lords Report 86-I (Session 2004-05), Paragraph 231

assumed that they have strongly-held views on a matter. These figures may well, therefore, provide an illustration of the balance of committed opinion on the subject. They also align closely, I have to say, with my own experience of talking to a wide range of people - that, while there is a core of decided opinion on each side of the debate, there is a large constituency (perhaps between a half and two thirds) in between with no firmly-held or thought-out view in the matter but willing to sign up to what sounds decent and compassionate.

Knowledge of the Subject

We are looking here at a very complex subject. The question of whether 'assisted dying' should be legalised is one that transcends a number of fields of knowledge and expertise, including the law, medical practice, mental health, ethics and the experience of those jurisdictions around the world that have chosen to go down the 'assisted dying' road. Most of us lead busy lives. We have neither the time nor, in many cases, the inclination to acquire serious knowledge of more than a handful of subjects that are of immediate concern to us. Whether we care to admit it or not, we are dependent for our perceptions of most of the issues of the day on what we read in newspapers and see or hear on television or radio. I have views on such things as the world economy, global warming and crime, but I cannot in all honesty claim that they are evidence-based views deriving from careful and dispassionate analysis of the facts.

There is also a lack of understanding among some people about what 'assisted dying' actually means. I have encountered people who think that legalising 'assisted dying' means permitting them to refuse or discontinue life-prolonging treatment. When I have pointed out to them that this is already legal and that 'assisted dying' is about providing lethal drugs for people to take their own lives, the information has been met with surprise.

Media reporting, moreover, tends to focus on the exceptional or the unusual. We hear of the occasional air disaster but not of the hundreds of thousands of safe landings that occur every year. Health care scandals make the front page but the tens of thousands of successful operations and treatments that are carried out go unacknowledged. What happens to most of us most of the time just isn't news.

There is also an increasing tendency in the media to focus on human-interest stories rather than on careful analysis of the facts. As Professor Clive Seale noted a few years ago:

> *"Journalists like to show ordinary people behaving like heroes and being 'victims' in need of rescue, in this case from the deterioration of their own bodies and from those who will not accede to requests for assisted dying, who are thereby constituted as 'villains'"*[5].

We can easily relate such stories to our own lives and ask ourselves whether the same thing could happen to us. But they can give us a distorted picture of what life is really like. Take, for instance, journeys by Britons to end their lives at the Dignitas assisted suicide facility in Switzerland. These are rare events - in 2016 0.008 per cent of deaths of Britons took this form. To say this is not to make light of these deaths. Every death, from whatever cause and in whatever manner, is a matter for sober reflection and respect. A death at Dignitas attracts media attention because such deaths are unusual. But the resultant publicity can easily create the false perception that such journeys are more numerous than in fact they are and fuel beliefs that the law in this country is in need of change.

---

[5] Seale. C. (2010) 'How the Mass Media Report Social Statistics: A Case Study
Concerning Research on End-of-Life Decisions', *Social Science and Medicine*. 71, pp.
861–8.

There are some, on both sides of the debate, who appear to see legalisation of 'assisted dying' as just one element of a wider package of social legislation and they adopt positions for or against legalisation by reference to the views they hold on other issues. This bulk-buy approach to legislating is misguided. Intelligent people should not be buying their opinions on issues of the day as a job lot. Attempts by supporters and opponents of legalised assisted suicide to hitch their wagons to other causes do not help the debate on this complex and emotive subject. We should be examining each social issue as it comes forward on its own merits and with regard to the evidence surrounding it rather than just asking ourselves whether it fits neatly with the opinions we already hold on other subjects.

In Conclusion

It is impossible to understand the 'assisted dying' debate without an awareness of the social changes that have taken place since the end of the Second World War and without an appreciation of the pressures under which seriously ill people now live. As a society we have turned our backs on death and dying: they are things which we know are inevitable but which increasingly we put out of our minds and the management of which we delegate to professionals. We have come to see choice and control as central features of the good life.

At the same time we are living longer lives but this longevity is not always matched by the health we once enjoyed. Modern medicine may be able to postpone our dying but the extended life it provides is not always congenial and in some cases can involve distress. Family support for the elderly and the sick cannot any longer be taken for granted.

This social perspective is important because the proposals for legalisation that are being placed before us are being linked with serious illness and presented as something that should be part of medical practice. In reality, this is primarily a social rather than a medical issue.

CHAPTER FOUR

AS LIFE DRAWS TO A CLOSE

ILORA FINLAY

The way a person dies lives in the memory of those left behind

We are all going to die – every year in Britain around 500,000 of us do – and many of us will die after a period of incurable illness. It has been estimated[1] that around three quarters of those who die will have a palliative phase to their illness. This is the role of doctors and nurses who are trained in palliative care - a branch of medicine for which Britain is internationally recognised. In a recent Economist Intelligence Unit survey of the quality of the dying experience Britain was rated in top place out of eighty nations[2].

Origins

It was not always like this. Even as late as the mid-twentieth century dying was often painful and distressing both for the patient and for his or her family to witness. The late Dame Cicely Saunders, internationally regarded as the founder of the modern hospice movement, observed that how people die remains in the memory of those who live on. Cicely Saunders initially trained in

---

[1] Etkind, S.N., Bone, A.E., Gomes, B. *et al.* How many people will need palliative care in 2040? Past trends, future projections and implications for services. *BMC Med* **15,** 102 (2017). https://doi.org/10.1186/s12916-017-0860-2

[2] The 2015 Quality of Death Index, Ranking Palliative Care Across the World, The Economist Intelligence Unit

social work, then in nursing before going on to train as a doctor. The mission she set herself was to improve care at the end of life. It was the middle of the last century, and she saw terrible dying all around her. Inspired by one of her patients, she raised funds for and opened St Christopher's Hospice in the 1960s, determined that strong research evidence would underpin the changes she knew had to happen. She pioneered the treatment of pain, describing 'total pain' and its management. This recognised that the relief of physical pain is only part of pain relief. Her research had shown that social, psychological, emotional and spiritual pain interact with and exacerbate the experience of physiological pain. She showed the world that each patient must be seen and treated as a whole, not simply as a collection of physical symptoms.

Cicely's and her colleagues' research revolutionised the practice of analgesia, which until then had been riven with ignorance. They pioneered the administration of morphine by mouth, bringing relief to millions, and the use of morphine in a variety of doses fitted to the needs of each individual patient rather than the one-size-fits-all approach that had been often followed in the past. The modern hospice movement was built on this work. By the late twentieth century hospices were shedding their image of places where people went to die and becoming recognised not just for care in the last days of life but also, as today, places where incurably ill people go to have difficult symptoms treated by experts and their medical care re-set before returning to the community.

What is Palliative Care?

Palliative care comprises two main elements. One is generalist care, which is core palliative care provided by clinicians who have had some training in the discipline, such as general practitioners and district nurses, medical and surgical teams in hospitals, and nurses in many nursing homes. The other element is specialist care, provided by those who have had specialist training. They are usually called in when difficult problems arise, beyond the skills and experience of the generalist services, and are able to provide assistance, working with and supporting the generalist teams who are usually delivering the main elements of care. The level of palliative care varies from patient to patient and an important task is to identify the individual needs of each one and to tailor the treatment accordingly.

Palliative care can be provided anywhere. It is not confined to hospices. Specialists also reach out into the community, working alongside primary care. They may have intensive involvement if patients particularly wish to remain in their own homes at all stages of their final illness. In hospitals, specialist palliative care teams provide expert advice and treatment and are often to be found working in parallel with or integrated with other departments.

Care in hospices embodies both general and specialist care and is led by specialists in the science and art of palliative care. Many hospices provide hospice-at-home support as well as in-patient or day-hospice services, and palliative care specialists in hospitals in many cases also provide care in hospices. Through this interweaving web of specialists and generalists, research and educational initiatives are constantly driving up the standards of all and moving forward the knowledge and experience base of this relatively new discipline.

It is important to understand that palliative care is not just something for people who are terminally ill and approaching death. While many of the services provided are for people who are nearing the end of their lives, palliative care is there for those with incurable conditions, some of which (for example, heart disease or multiple sclerosis) can be life-shortening but careful management of which can enable the patient to live well for an extended period of time.

The World Health Organisation (WHO) defines palliative care as:

> *"an approach that improves the quality of life of patients and their families facing the problem associated with life-threatening illness, through the prevention and relief of suffering by means of early identification and impeccable assessment and treatment of pain and other problems, physical, psychosocial and spiritual[3]".*

According to the WHO, palliative care:

- *"provides relief from pain and other distressing symptoms;*
- *affirms life and regards dying as a normal process;*
- *intends neither to hasten or postpone death;*
- *integrates the psychological and spiritual aspects of patient care;*
- *offers a support system to help patients live as actively as possible until death;*
- *offers a support system to help the family cope during the patient's illness and in their own bereavement;*
- *uses a team approach to address the needs of patients and their families, including bereavement counselling, if indicated;*
- *will enhance quality of life, and may also positively influence the course of illness;*
- *is applicable early in the course of illness, in conjunction with other therapies that are intended to prolong life, such as chemotherapy or radiation therapy, and includes those investigations needed to better understand and manage distressing clinical complications".*

Palliative Care in the United Kingdom

In 1989 palliative care was recognised by the Royal College of Physicians as a separate branch of medicine requiring specialist training. In the early days those entering palliative care had come from other medical specialities or from general practice. For the last 30 years a four-year training programme has been mandatory for doctors to be recognised as specialists in palliative care. Other branches of medicine receive some training in this area. For

[3] https://www.who.int/cancer/palliative/definition/en/

example, core training in palliative care is provided in medical schools, in training for general practice and in some other disciplines, such as geriatric medicine or oncology, where the need for such skills might arise. But the cutting edge of the science of palliative care is to be found in hospices and specialist teams in hospitals. This situation is not reflected in many parts of the world, where training is more rudimentary and palliative care is not a recognised medical specialty. In palliative care it is no exaggeration to say that Britain leads the world.

Palliative care is not a course of treatment similar to the administration of antibiotics or the performance of surgery. Its recipients are incurably ill and, while other treatments may take place in parallel, palliative care is designed to give effective relief to the symptoms of the underlying illness, to detect and treat any reversible incidental conditions that may be causing distress and to enable the patient to live as near normal a life as possible. This demands meticulous attention to detail, with frequent treatment reviews and adjustments to medication. A major part of this is the relief of physiological pain but palliative care also includes the relief of psychosocial and emotional distress as well as paying attention to the needs of the family who are facing bereavement, particularly where children face loss.

The science of pain relief has come a long way since the middle of the twentieth century. In those days, for example, there was widespread ignorance of the proper use of drugs such as morphine. There was no understanding that it could be given by mouth or that doses could and should be titrated up to achieve pain control. In the past fixed doses, which were often inadequate to provide lasting pain relief, were injected into muscles, which was painful. Predictable side-effects, such as constipation or nausea, were ignored rather than anticipated and appropriate preventive action taken. As a result, large numbers of dying people did not receive adequate analgesia as well as having to endure drug-induced side-effects. Close links with anaesthetic pain departments in some parts of the UK have made spinal, epidural and other nerve block techniques available for relief of some relatively rare complex pain syndromes.

Today patients can take morphine and other opioids by mouth and, where appropriate, in larger doses in such a way that the patient is not only relieved of pain but also remains fully alert and able to be active - in some cases, to return to work. It is also known that there are some types of pain, such as pain from damaged nerve pathways (known as neuropathic pain), that do not respond well to morphine and need other medications. Some pain, such as cancer bone pain, responds well to a targeted dose of radiotherapy. As always, the accurate diagnosis of the underlying cause of each pain needs to be meticulous if it is to guide the appropriate therapy.

An important element of pain relief is knowledge of the levels at which individual drugs or combinations of drugs will provide effective pain relief without exceeding the toxic threshold. This requires that doctors identify the correct level of pain relief for each individual patient and maintain that level with analgesic drugs or combinations of drugs without causing undesirable side effects or exceeding the toxic threshold. Analgesia is not a one-size-fits-all activity. It can vary from patient to patient and the palliative care physician's task is to identify accurately what is needed and to provide the necessary relief in each individual case without harming the patient.

Excessive administration of opioids can be fatal by depressing the respiratory system, and the myth is occasionally heard that doctors hasten patients' deaths by this means. These fears were not helped by the revelations surrounding the case of Dr Harold Shipman, a GP who was convicted early in this century of killing patients through the administration of morphine overdoses. Shipman was a mass murderer using the cover of his professional identity to perpetrate his crimes. It need hardly be said that hastening patients' deaths is anathema to modern medicine and especially to palliative care. In fact, the fall-out from the Shipman case has had the unintended consequence of making many physicians, who are anxious not be mistakenly accused of malpractice, ultra-cautious about prescribing morphine or increasing dosages where this is needed for proper pain relief.

Physiological pain relief is, however, only part of the role of modern palliative care. As observed above, Cicely Saunders identified what she referred to as 'total pain'. Pain feels worse if a patient is frightened, anxious or isolated in a black hole of despair. Palliative care services therefore involve not only doctors and nurses trained in physiological pain relief but also psychologists, psychiatrists, social workers and others who have skills to contribute to the identification and relief of the patient's whole suffering.

Palliative care grew out of cancer care, as cancer was a condition which was almost always fatal and could involve considerable suffering. This history continues to be reflected even today, when hospices and palliative care teams in hospitals see more patients diagnosed with cancer than patients with other conditions.

However, that situation is changing. As longevity has increased with advances in medical and surgical care, so we are seeing more cases of incurable illness associated with other conditions which are often, though not invariably, associated with ageing and which can have relatively-long trajectories between diagnosis and death. Parkinson's disease, motor neurone disease, heart disease and dementia are examples. At the same time breakthroughs in the early diagnosis and treatment of many forms of cancer have led to patients with these conditions going into remission and having extended life spans. All this means that the work of palliative care is broadening its remit to meet the needs of those dying of a wide variety of life-limiting conditions.

At the same time palliative care doctors and nurses have been making a major contribution to the care of patients suffering from the effects of Covid-19. The discipline was catapulted to the fore with the onset of the pandemic and has worked alongside, and integrated with, acute medical and intensive care teams. Palliative care input has been shown to be essential, and morphine and other medications have been used judiciously to bring symptom relief to many of those dying of Covid-19. In the post-pandemic world this transformation must be maintained, with palliative care more fully integrated into health care systems and with early involvement of specialists when distress is not rapidly coming under control.

Availability

However, if this is to be achieved, there is a need for greater investment in specialist palliative care. I have mentioned above that Britain has been ranked in first place among eighty nations, including all major Western countries, for the quality of its end of life care. When it comes to quantity, the story is not quite so favourable. In 2016-17 there were just 628 consultants in palliative medicine across the whole of the UK, over half of whom were working less than full time.[4] This contrasts with a projected need of around double that number. The availability of such expert services varies from region to region, with some areas having more ready access to specialist treatment in hospitals or hospices than others. It is not too wide of the mark to talk of a postcode lottery.

Part of the problem is that palliative care has tended to be something of a Cinderella among health services. Though we will all die one day and many of us will need expert support in our last weeks or months of life, palliative care's successes – which are considerable – attract little attention in the media. The sad fact is

[4] https://www.rcpmedicalcare.org.uk/developing-physicians/specialties/palliative-medicine/workforce (accessed 1/7/20)

that care of the dying lacks the glamour of surgical or medical breakthroughs, even though these latter may benefit fewer people than those in need of modern palliative care. If this unhappy situation is to be corrected, there is need for better resourcing of the discipline. Earlier diagnosis of incurable illness and referral for palliative care would make a huge difference to outcomes for patients.

Another factor of uneven distribution of services is the dependence of hospices on donations and public subscriptions for the greater part of their income. Anyone who has visited a hospice cannot fail to appreciate the skills and devotion of the staff, the expert treatment they provide and the calm and reassuring atmosphere that they create for those who come to them, whether for day or in-patient care. Hospices in relatively prosperous parts of the country are often, though not invariably, better placed than others in less well-heeled areas. Some hospices cannot afford to employ a full-time medical director but have to call in general practitioners with a special interest in hospice care on a part-time basis. These doctors will have undergone some additional training in the discipline and increasingly hospice doctors at all grades are coming together in local networks to share knowledge and experience.

Nor should we overlook the palliative care that is provided in the community by dedicated doctors and nurses visiting very seriously ill patients in their homes. They have often undergone additional training in palliative care and provide excellent personalised care. But there can be failures sometimes to refer patients for specialist attention early enough and out-of-hours support is not always available to families struggling to care for relatives dying at home. As a result, dying patients can all too often find themselves rushed into Accident and Emergency Units and may die separated from their loved ones. Surveys show that most of us would wish to die in our homes rather than in hospital. If that is to become a reality, there is a need for better 24-hour availability of palliative care services in the community, for better care planning to ensure just-in-case medication is available so that families are not hunting for an open pharmacy at nights or weekends, and for improved liaison between community services and specialist teams.

When death comes...

Most dying patients whom palliative care specialists encounter describe a sense of being ready to let go and of an inner calm. Some are fearful of what lies ahead, usually when they have not had open and honest conversations with those providing care, as many fear things that are extremely unlikely to happen. Fear of the unknown can be lessened when that fear is spoken about openly and plans put in place to mitigate all eventualities. That fear may be existential, of feeling a need to make sense of our lives, or it may be rooted in anguish over personal relationships, or it may be fear of dying in pain or of suffocating. It can also stem from an experience of having watched a loved one die many years before and of having misread what was happening. Most doctors who care for dying patients have come across the anguished relative who is convinced that the dying person with whom they are sitting is in pain or otherwise distressed, when the patient is in fact dying peacefully.

Palliative care consultant Dr Kathryn Mannix has described such a scene in an anonymised account of the death of a 78-year-old widow, whom she has called Cara and who is dying at home of cancer. Two of her children, Dulcie and Ira, are at her bedside. A palliative care nurse has explained to them how their mother's dying will occur and what signs to look for. Cara sleeps more and more as death approaches, waking periodically.

> *"Cara's breathing is changing. She no longer wakes up when her family call her name; the nurses have noticed that her hands and feet are feeling cool as her circulation begins to shut down. Sometimes she takes a deeper breath and makes a noisy exhalation, as the palliative care nurse had predicted.*

"Dulcie sits beside her Mum and holds her hand, talking to her gently about funny incidents from their home life together and telling stories about the grandchildren. She is glad to see her Mum looking so peaceful.

"Ira paces the room, saying 'You wouldn't let a dog suffer like this!' Each time Cara takes a deep breath he says 'See! She's in pain.' Ira believes his Mum is suffering unbearably.

"And yet both are witnessing the same death"[5]

Unfamiliarity with the process of dying is, as observed in an earlier chapter[6], a growing problem. It predisposes us to regard death as an agonising process, whereas in the great majority of cases that is not so. None of us really knows what dying is like until it is our turn to do so, but the clear experience of those of us who have spent our lives caring for the dying suggests that it is more a process of relaxing and letting go.

Surprisingly, things can change dramatically as death draws near. There is the phenomenon that I have often seen in those near death, which I would colloquially describe as 'the rise before the fall' – when a dying patient regains surprising and unexpected energy before gently dying. I have seen events that no one could ever have thought would happen – a wedding enjoyed or a special evening with the family before death arrives gently and peacefully. It is as if that was the last task in life that often came as a great surprise to the family. Often families in acute bereavement describe their astonishment at the unexpected and important conversations that have opened up between them and dying relatives at the last moments and that have left them with valuable memories to treasure for the rest of their lives. And sometimes it has been a gentle smile or a last loving look as the person lets go of life, knowing those they love were prepared for this parting.

---

[5] 'What Happens When We Die?', Dr Kathryn Mannix, Living and Dying Well

[6] See Chapter Three

To anticipate such situations, palliative care needs to be involved as soon as it looks as though a terminally ill patient is entering his or her final illness. Fears have to be tackled head on rather than brushed aside. A clear plan must be drawn up and discussed honestly with patients and their families. Some years ago I had under my care a dying man whom I will call John. Like his father, who had died some years before him, he had been a smoker and, also like his father, he was now dying of lung cancer. His bone pain had been brought under control by a combination of radiotherapy and regular doses of slow-release morphine. But the image of his father, breathless and on oxygen, haunted him.

John needed to know that any breathlessness that he might experience would be a priority for us to relieve. He needed to know that any fluid around his lung would be removed rapidly, that his morphine dose could be varied and other drugs introduced to overcome his breathlessness, that his good lung would keep working and that he wouldn't suffocate. He needed to know that the physiotherapist would show him how to do more without precipitating breathlessness. And, above all, he needed to know whom to call, day or night, if he were to find himself in distress, that his dying would come as he became weaker and more tired and that he would slip into a coma and die gently and peacefully, confident that he would not die as he felt his father had done. When John had had all this explained to him, he became calmer and in due course he died peacefully.

Palliative care is not a panacea. There are cases which challenge even the most expert of us. Often these are instances where there has been a failure to involve specialist care in a sufficiently timely manner or where the natural and relievable suffering of dying is compounded by deep-seated fear or despair. It is undeniable, however, that in Britain, and increasingly in other countries, medical science is able to relieve the suffering of dying in a way that would have been unimaginable two or three generations ago. If we are to capitalise on these breakthroughs, we need better resourcing and more joined-up working. As I observed at the outset of this chapter, we are all of us going to die one day.

Palliative Care and 'Assisted Dying'

Those who advocate legalisation of 'assisted dying' assure us that they support the provision of good palliative care services and that legalising the supply of lethal drugs to terminally ill patients is not an alternative but an addition to palliative care. The parliamentary bills they have sponsored at Westminster include provision that a person seeking 'assisted dying' should have been *"fully informed of the palliative, hospice and other care which is available"*[7].

However, there is a fundamental difference between being briefed on the relief that palliative care can bring and experiencing that relief. Nor is it made clear who is to provide such a briefing – a specialist in palliative care? or a generalist doctor who may or may not be up to date with the latest state of the art? A briefing by a specialist might not be such a straightforward proposition as it might seem at first sight. In a 2019 survey by the Royal College of Physicians, only 4.8 per cent of palliative medicine specialists stated that they would be prepared to participate in 'assisted dying' if the law were to be changed.

The central problem here is that care of the dying, like dying itself, is a complex matter that cannot be managed by the tick-in-the-box approach or the one-off consultation that these parliamentary bills envisage. While I do not therefore doubt the sincerity of those who see 'assisted dying' as an adjunct to palliative care, such an approach is over-simplistic and fails to recognise the dynamic relationship between patient and clinical team in those who are very ill.

[7] See, for example, HL Bill 69 (Session 2020-21), Section 3(4)

In Conclusion

Palliative care in Britain is a highly-developed branch of medicine, unlike in many other countries including those that have gone down the 'assisted dying' road. Over the last 50 years it has been at the heart of a revolution in care of the incurably ill and the dying. Distressing deaths still occur but they are a small faction today of what they were in the middle of the twentieth century and advances in the science are being made year by year.

Sadly, the high quality of palliative care in Britain is not always matched by its nationwide availability. Better resourcing is needed in order to ensure that all incurably ill people are able to access high-quality palliative care when they need it, wherever they live and at whatever time of day or night. This is in many respects key to meeting the wish of the majority of patients to die in their own homes rather than in hospital.

Early identification of the need for specialist palliative care is essential. If, as sometimes happens, it is called upon only in the last days or weeks of life when someone has been ill for months, patients will have been denied much that could have been done to improve their quality of life. It is time for palliative care expertise to be recognised as an essential part of the process of caring for all who are dying rather than as an optional extra for some. We are all going to die and most of us will need palliative care in one form or another as we do.

Palliative care is not a one-off event, a one-size-fits-all treatment or a briefing. It is an ongoing process of specialised care for people who face incurable and life threatening or life-limiting illness. It is not unusual for patients who have had good palliative care to say they would not have believed the transformation it has brought to their lives if they had not experienced it.

As the late Dame Cicely Saunders said, the way a person dies lives on in the memory of those left behind. Perceptions of how our grandparents died in previous decades, combined with a widespread and growing lack of familiarity with the process of dying, is undoubtedly a factor in creating a fear of dying and support for 'assisted dying'. It is time to set the record straight.

Chapter Five

What News from Abroad?

Robert Preston

The wise learn from the experience of others

What is being called 'assisted dying' comes in two main forms – physician-assisted suicide (PAS), where a doctor supplies lethal drugs for self-administration to a requesting patient; and physician-administered euthanasia (PAE), where a doctor administers lethal drugs directly to such a patient.

PAS laws have been enacted in a small number of the fifty US States, including Oregon, Washington State, Vermont, California, Colorado and Hawaii - plus Washington DC. There have been court rulings to the effect that it is permissible under existing legislation in one or two other States. Assisted suicide is also legal in Switzerland, though as an exception to the Penal Code rather than as the result of legislation licensing such acts.

PAE has been legalised in The Netherlands[1], Belgium and Luxembourg. In 2015 a law permitting PAE was enacted in the Canadian Province of Quebec. This was followed in 2016 by a federal law permitting both PAE and PAS in Canada's other Provinces and Territories. This latter law, known as 'Medical Assistance in Dying' (MAiD), followed a ruling by the Canadian

---

[1] In The Netherlands both physician-assisted suicide and physician-administered euthanasia have been legalised

Supreme Court that the existing law's prohibition was in conflict with Section 7 of the Canadian Charter of Rights and Freedoms[2].

In this chapter I examine the experience of two of these jurisdictions, Oregon and The Netherlands, which are representative of the two different approaches - PAS (Oregon) and PAE (Netherlands). They are also the jurisdictions where there is the most published evidence of how such legislation is turning out in practice. In addition, I offer a brief description of the situation in Canada in so far as that can be ascertained at this moment. It is not possible at the time of going to press to provide more than an outline picture and a provisional assessment of Canada's MAiD law. This is partly because the legislation there is of relatively recent enactment - and is undergoing some amendment - and partly because there is a shortage of published official data on how MAiD is turning out.

Also included is a short section on assisted suicide in Switzerland. The Swiss system has not so far been seen by advocates of 'assisted dying' as a model for legislation but it is worth looking at because of the different approach that it employs.

Oregon[3]

What the law says

For the purposes of the current political debate in England, Wales and Scotland, Oregon may be regarded as the most relevant model. Indeed, it is held up to us by campaigners for legalisation here as an example of good practice. Oregon's PAS law was passed in 1994. It was the result of a Citizens' Initiative, which means that it was proposed by individuals rather than by the State Government.

---

[2] Carter *v.* Canada (Attorney General), 2015 SCC 5 (6 February 2015)

[3] In relation to this section, see also 'Physician-Assisted Suicide – A Clean Bill of Health', by the author and published in the British Medical Bulletin 13 July 2017

Oregon's Death with Dignity Act (DWDA), as it is called, permits doctors to prescribe lethal drugs for terminally ill patients who are considered to have a prognosis of life remaining of six months or less and who are thought to be mentally competent and acting voluntarily. Where a request is approved, the doctor's role is limited to the writing of a prescription for lethal drugs: there is no requirement on the doctor to oversee the act of suicide or to be present when the drugs are swallowed. When the prescription is dispensed, the patient takes the drugs home and either ingests them or stores them for possible future use.

A doctor who writes a prescription for lethal drugs is required by law to notify the Oregon Health Authority (OHA). The OHA collects the reports from doctors and checks them to ensure that all the required information has been provided and that there is no apparent irregularity. In the latter event, the report in question may be passed to the Oregon Medical Board (the equivalent of the General Medical Council in Britain) for consideration. The OHA uses the reports from doctors as a basis for preparing annual reports on the working of the law. The first such report was published in 1998. At the time of writing 22 such reports are available.

The Reports

The reports are essentially statistical analyses. By this I mean that they focus on how many people have died under the terms of the DWDA, what medical conditions they had, how old they were, how long they had known the prescribing doctors, how many of them had been referred for psychiatric assessment and so on. They tell us little about how requests for PAS are being handled. This approach contrasts, as we will see, with that of The Netherlands, whose annual reports not only give the reader data about the incidence of PAS and PAE but also discuss issues which have arisen and provide some anonymised case summaries to illustrate how specific aspects of the assessment process have been handled.

Numbers

The graph on Page 77 shows the incidence of physician-assisted suicide in Oregon from 1998 to 2019. The rise in numbers of deaths has not been uniform: there have been ups and downs between individual years. The overall trend, however, has been upwards. As a proportion of total deaths in Oregon the numbers are small: in 2019 out of every 10,000 deaths in Oregon 51.9 resulted from ingestion of lethal drugs under the DWDA. On the other hand, the number of such deaths in 2019 was almost twelve times the number in the first year of the law's operation (1998).

There were 188 recorded DWDA deaths in 2019. Though that number may look small, it has to be remembered that Oregon is a sparsely-populated State: its total population is less than half that of Greater London. Oregon's 2019 death rate from PAS is the equivalent of around 2,800 such assisted suicide deaths annually in England and Wales if a similar law, with a similar death rate, were to apply here. On the same basis a law like Oregon's in Scotland could be expected to result in 200 to 300 PAS deaths a year.

In every year since the DWDA came into force there were more prescriptions for lethal drugs issued than deaths resulting. This is because some recipients take the drugs home and keep them for use at a later date and some of them do not ingest the drugs at all but die of natural causes. The number of deaths in any one year therefore includes people who have received lethal drugs in earlier years but postponed taking them. This introduces a complication into the recording of data. The OHA annual reports record those deaths during the year of which the Authority has been informed but notes also the number of prescriptions issued where 'ingestion status' is unknown - ie it is not known whether or not the drugs have been ingested during the year in question. Thus, for example, the OHA tells us that, in addition to 170 people who received lethal drugs in 2019 and used them to end their lives during that year, another 18 people died in that year after receiving prescriptions for

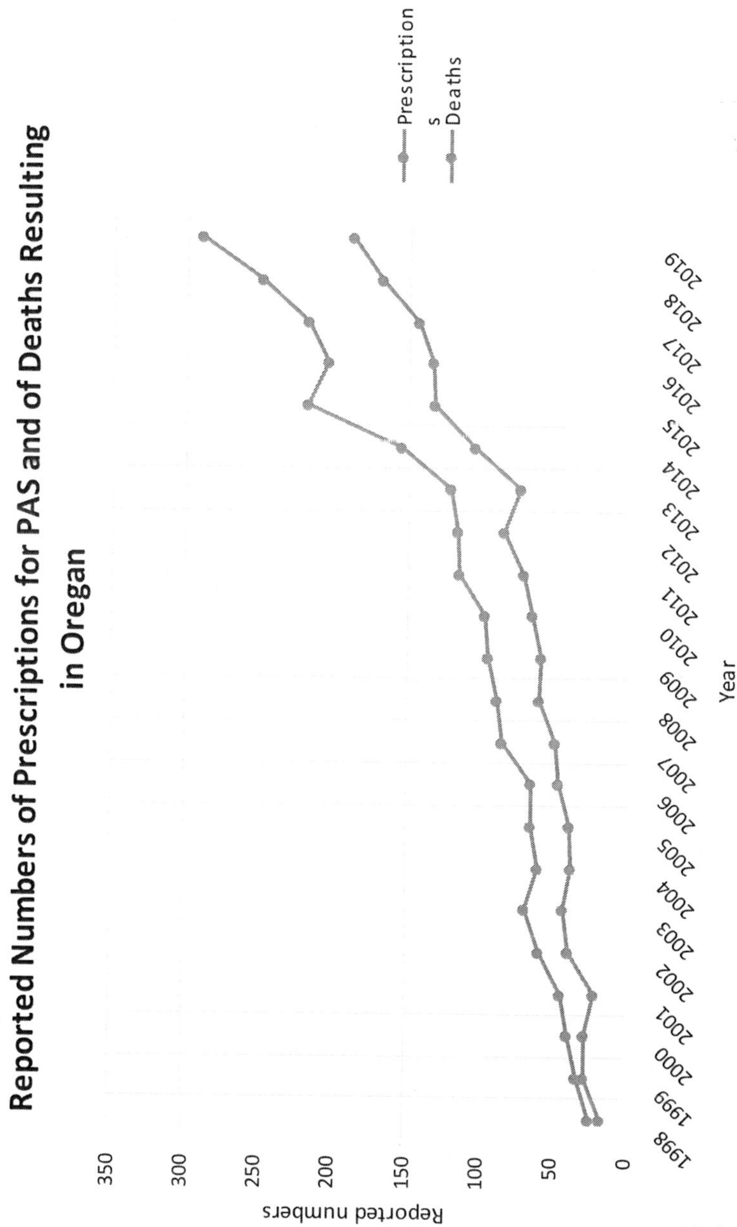
Reported Numbers of Prescriptions for PAS and of Deaths Resulting in Oregan
Reported numbers
350
300
250
200
150
100
50
0
1998
1999
2000
2001
2002
2003
2004
2005
2006
2007
2008
2009
2010
2011
2012
2013
2014
2015
2016
2017
2018
2019
Year
Prescriptions
Deaths

lethal drugs in previous years and that, in addition, there were 58 recipients of drugs in 2019 whose 'ingestion status' was pending or unknown. Some of these can be expected to appear in the numbers of DWDA deaths recorded in future years.

Characteristics

The 2019 report tells us that over the period from 1998 to 2019 59.0 per cent of those who died by PAS were male and 41.0 per cent female. 74.5 per cent were aged 65 or over, with the median age being 74. 96.3 per cent were white; 48.9 per cent were married, 17.6 per cent widowed and 20.7 per cent divorced. 53.0 per cent had been educated to bachelors degree or above, while only 8.0 per cent had had an education that was below high school graduate level. 89.9 per cent were enrolled in hospice care programmes and nearly all were covered by private or state health care insurance.

68.1 per cent of those who ended their lives under the DWDA had been suffering from cancer and 13.8 per cent had had neurological disorders, in most cases amyotrophic lateral sclerosis (known in Britain as motor neurone disease). The remainder had been suffering from a range of illnesses including respiratory disease, heart/circulatory disease, gastro-intestinal disease and what the report calls 'other illnesses'.

Only one (0.5 per cent) of those who died by physician-assisted suicide under the DWDA had been referred for psychiatric assessment. This very low referral figure needs to be treated with some caution. It does not mean that only 0.5 per cent of those who requested lethal drugs were referred for psychiatric assessment but that 0.5 per cent of those who were judged ultimately to have capacity had been so referred. It may well be (the reports do not tell us) that in cases where requests were turned down the rate of referral was higher.

94.1 per cent died at home. The prescribing doctor was present at the death in less than 1 in 5 cases. The median length of the doctor-patient relationship was 14 weeks within a range of 0 to 1,220 weeks. The median length of time between the first request for physician-assisted suicide and the death of the person making the request was 45 days within a range of 15 to 1,503 days.

The most commonly-cited reasons given for ending life under the DWDA were *"less able to engage in activities making life enjoyable"* (90.4 per cent) and *"losing autonomy"* (86.7 per cent). Inadequate pain control or concern about it came well down the list at 33.0 per cent. 59.0 per cent cited being a burden on family, friends or caregivers.

Issues

Considered as statistical data the reports are valuable. They do not, however, shed much light on the quality of the process by which requests for PAS are being considered in Oregon. For example, they tell us nothing about the length or nature of the consultations that are taking place between those who request lethal drugs under the DWDA and the doctors who consider those requests. Was a doctor's agreement given on the basis of a single consultation? Or was it the culmination of a series of consultations over a period of time? Did the doctor talk with the applicants' relatives or with others who knew the applicant well? What steps did the doctor take to establish whether the request represented a settled wish or whether there was any undue influence at work in the background or whether an applicant was seeking to remove him- or herself as a perceived burden on others rather than because of a heartfelt personal wish to die? On these and other questions the reports are silent. Yet they are vitally important questions that need to be answered if we are to be able to reach an objective view of whether Oregon's law is protecting vulnerable people.

Heightened Risk

In the absence of such qualitative reporting we have to make inferences from the data provided and to look at research into specific topics carried out by individuals or groups. There have been a number of these latter. One of the most commonly cited by advocates of legalisation is a study[4] the results of which were published in 2007 and which concluded that there was "*no evidence of heightened risk*" to various groups of people including the elderly, women, the uninsured, people of low educational attainment, poor people, racial and ethnic minorities, people with physical disabilities and non-terminal illnesses, minors and people suffering from depression. It concluded:

> "*We found no evidence to justify the grave and important concern often expressed about the potential for abuse - namely, the fear that legalised physician-assisted dying will target the vulnerable or pose the greatest risk to people in vulnerable groups*"

These are impressive findings - or they would be if they could be substantiated. Closer inspection, however, raises questions about the study's methodology.

For example, the study found that "*persons aged 18-64 years were over three times more likely than those over age 85 years to receive assisted dying*". On this basis it concluded that there was no evidence of heightened risk from Oregon's law to elderly people. However, this finding took no account of people aged between 65 and 84, a group whom most people would regard as elderly. This is an inexplicable omission, as the official annual reports show that people in the 65-84 age group account for the majority of those who have ended their lives under Oregon's law since 1997. If they are included, a different picture emerges.

---

[4] Legal physician-assisted dying in Oregon and the Netherlands: evidence concerning the impact on patients in 'vulnerable' groups. Battin, MP et al, Journal of Medical Ethics 2007; 33: 591-597

Or, again, the study concluded that, as women were not more likely than men to resort to physician-assisted suicide, they too were not at heightened risk; and that, as requests for assisted suicide originated more frequently from people with health insurance or with high educational attainment, there was no heightened risk to the poor or to people of low educational status.

These conclusions may well be correct but their relevance is open to question. As was pointed out in an article[5] reviewing the results of the research, vulnerability in end-of-life decision-making is more related to such things as temperament, communicative abilities, personal problems, inadequate medical treatment or loss of self-worth than to traditional socio-economic factors such as gender, income or race. Even these latter have been interpreted in a questionable manner. For example, having established that 'college graduates' were 7.6 times more likely to die from physician-assisted suicide than were those without a high school diploma, the researchers concluded that people of low educational status were not at heightened risk from the DWDA. That may possibly be so, but the researchers do not seem to have reflected that perhaps the better-educated might themselves be at heightened risk of ending their lives through legalised assisted suicide. Vulnerability is something to which we are all susceptible, albeit in different ways. It is not an exclusive preserve of the poor or the less-well-educated.

Depression

The same study conceded that "*not all patients who requested assistance were specifically evaluated by mental health professionals*" and that, "*because many cases of depression are missed in primary*

[5] Legal physician-assisted suicide in Oregon and The Netherlands: evidence concerning the impact on patients in vulnerable groups - another perspective on Oregon's data, Finlay, I and George, R, Journal of Medical Ethics 2011; 37:171-174

care, it is possible that some depressed patients received lethal prescriptions". But, it concluded, "*there is no direct evidence that depressed patients are at higher risk for receiving assistance in dying under the ODDA*[6]*".*

This conclusion became more difficult to justify a year later when another study[7] found evidence that some people suffering from undiagnosed clinical depression had indeed ended their lives with lethal drugs supplied to them by doctors under the DWDA. The researchers had examined the case files of a small number of people who had requested physician-assisted suicide and they considered to what extent depression had been a factor in their requests. It reported:

> "*42 patients died by the end of the study; 18 received a prescription for a lethal drug under the Death with Dignity Act and nine died by lethal ingestion. 15 participants who received a prescription for a lethal drug did not meet criteria for depression; three did. All three depressed participants died by lethal ingestion within two months of the research interview*".

In other words, one in six of a small sample of patients who died by PAS had been suffering from undiagnosed depression. The authors concluded:

> "*Although most terminally ill Oregonians who receive aid in dying do not have depressive disorders, the current practice of the Death with Dignity Act may fail to protect some patients whose choices are influenced by depression from receiving a prescription for a lethal drug*".

---

[6] ODDA = Oregon Death with Dignity Act (an alternative acronym to the DWDA)

[7] Prevalence of depression and anxiety in patients requesting physicians' aid in dying: cross sectional survey, Ganzini, L et al, British Medical Journal 2008; 337: a1682

Writing in 2014, the study's lead author, Oregon-based Professor of Psychiatry Linda Ganzini, said that:

> "*This finding supports the need for more active and systematic screening and surveillance for depression to determine which patients should be referred for mental health evaluation*"[8].

These findings cannot just be brushed aside by statements to the effect that a degree of sadness is to be expected in people who are terminally ill. There is indeed a distinction to be drawn between natural sadness and depression. But the question which this research raises is why doctors who agree to consider requests for physician-assisted suicide in Oregon are sometimes failing to detect the presence of clinical depression.

Professor Ganzini has shed some light on this question. She writes:

> "*Understanding whether depression influences the decision for PAD*[9] *requires knowing an individual over time while both depressed and euthymic. Ninety-five per cent of Oregon psychiatrists were somewhat or very confident in the context of a long-term relationship in which they could determine whether a mental disorder, such as depression, was influencing the decision for PAD; but only 6% were very confident that in a single evaluation they could make this assessment*"[10].

This brings us to an important aspect of the 'assisted dying' debate - the length of doctor-patient relationships.

Doctor-Patient Relationships

A long-term relationship does not in many cases seem to exist between people who request physician-assisted suicide under the

---

[8] Palliative Care and Ethics, Ed. Quill, TE and Miller FG, Oxford University Press 2014, Page 273.

[9] PAD = Physician-Assisted Dying (i.e. the supply of lethal drugs to terminally ill patients as permitted under Oregon's law)

[10] Ibid, Page 272.

DWDA and the doctors assessing them. Many doctors in Oregon are not willing to participate in these practices, with the result that some of those who request physician-assisted suicide have to find or to be introduced to doctors who are willing to consider their requests. Some of these referral doctors are writing prescriptions for lethal drugs for several patients. According to the OHA's most recent report, in 2019 one doctor wrote no fewer than 33 such prescriptions.

What we are looking at here is what has been called doctor-shopping. In 2019 the median length of the doctor-patient relationship for those who died by PAS was just fourteen weeks, in some cases just one week. Even where there has been a longer doctor-patient relationship there can be challenges in assessing how truly settled is a wish to die, whether the patient making the request is suffering from treatable depression and whether there could be anything in the patient's personal or domestic life that could be influencing the request. A doctor who has been selected solely in order to consider a request for physician-assisted suicide is ill-placed to make a knowledge-based assessment of this nature.

In Oregon the role of a doctor who agrees to consider a request for physician-assisted suicide ends when he or she has written a prescription for lethal drugs. The patient is then free to have the drugs dispensed by a pharmacist and to take them home either to ingest or to store for possible future use. Patients sometimes do not take the drugs at once and some never take them at all, regarding them as a form of insurance in case they find themselves in a position where they feel they cannot go on any longer. Whatever merit there may be in this practice, it raises a potential problem. Once the supply of drugs has been authorised, it is impossible to be sure that the person concerned does not come under pressure to take them or does not take them as the result a transient bout of depression or has not lost capacity before taking them. It is arguable therefore that, however vulnerable an applicant for lethal drugs may have been at the time of making the request, he or she could become more vulnerable having received them.

Prognosis

The DWDA requires that an applicant for PAS must be terminally ill and it defines terminal illness as "*an incurable and irreversible disease that has been medically confirmed and will, within reasonable medical judgement, produce death within six months".* It would appear, however, that this definition of terminal illness is not as restrictive as might appear at first sight. In 2017 Fabian Stahle, a Swedish researcher, contacted the OHA and asked whether the DWDA's criterion of terminal illness assumes that there will be no treatment given to manage or retard the patient's condition. According to Mr Stahle, the OHA confirmed that this was so[11]. This suggests that it is possible to qualify for a prescription for lethal drugs under the terms of the DWDA not only in a situation where a person is facing an unavoidable death within six months but also where someone has a chronic but treatable condition from which he or she will die within six months without treatment or medication. On this basis a person with a relatively common condition, such as (for example) insulin-dependent diabetes, could be classified as terminally ill and qualify for lethal drugs simply by declining or discontinuing the medication needed to manage the condition. To what extent deaths under the DWDA include such instances is not known. The published official data list numbers but they give no indication of the way in which doctors agreeing to supply lethal drugs have interpreted the requirement for an applicant to be terminally ill.

---

[11] https://drive.google.com/file/d/1xOZfLFrvuQcazZfFudEncpzp2b18NrUo/view

Voluntary Request

The DWDA requires that a request for lethal drugs should be made voluntarily. While this is an obvious requirement, its fulfilment is not as simple as might appear at first sight. The ability of a doctor to detect whether a request for lethal drugs may not be entirely voluntary but may stem from internal or external pressures or influences depends to a large extent on how well the doctor knows the patient, how many discussions of the request have taken place and what, if any, independent inquiries have been conducted.

The DWDA lays down no minimum requirements in this respect. It does not require a doctor considering a request to have known a requesting patient for any minimum length of time and it leaves the level of scrutiny to be applied to a request for lethal drugs to the doctor's discretion. In the words of the OHA report on Year 2017, *"it is up to the attending and consulting physicians to determine whether these requirements have been met".*

A doctor who has prescribed lethal drugs is required to report the fact to the OHA and to answer a number of questions by ticking a series of boxes. One of these is that the recipient of the drugs was judged to be acting voluntarily. Individual doctors may perhaps discuss requests in depth with those who make them and conduct searching inquiries to try to discover whether there are any internal or external pressures behind the request. But there is no requirement on them to deal with a request in that way.

Scrutiny

Speaking in the House of Lords in 2014, Lord Falconer stated[12] that "*there has been no evidence of abuse*" of Oregon's PAS law since its inception. The important word here is 'evidence'. A doctor who processes a request for physician-assisted suicide is required to report the fact to the OHA and to file a report of his (or her) action

[12] House of Lords Hansard, 18 July 2014, Col. 775

in the patient's medical record. The DWDA requires the OHA to "*review a sample of records maintained*" and to "*make rules to facilitate the collection of information regarding compliance with ORS 127.800 to 127.897*"[13]. But it adds that "*except as otherwise required by law, the information collected shall not be a public record and may not be made available for inspection by the public*"[14].

The Mackay Committee was told by the Oregon Department of Human Services[15] during a visit to Oregon in 2004 that its role in regard to the DWDA was limited:

> "*We are not a regulatory agency, at least not in this regard, so if we see that there are any problems that have happened, and there have been a number over the years, let us say that only one witness has signed or they did not wait 15 days*[16]*, our role is to report that to the Board of Medical Examiners*[17]*, which is the licensing board for physicians. We do not call the police or take away their licence, we are not regulatory in that regard*"[18].

The OHA's website confirms this limitation of its role. It states that "*the OHA does not investigate whether patients met the DWDA criteria, nor how their diagnosis, prognosis and treatment options were determined. OHA does not interpret the statute, other than the portion related to the reporting requirements. However, if any instances of non-compliance are found in the information received*

---

[13] 127.800 to 127.897 is the DWDA

[14] DWDA, 127.865, Section 3.11

[15] This Department at the time performed the monitoring role now discharged by the OHA.

[16] The DWDA requires a minimum of 15 days to elapse between the making of the first and second requests for physician-assisted suicide and a minimum of 48 hours between the making of a written request and the writing of a prescription for lethal drugs. However, see below under 'Waiting Period'.

[17] Now called the Oregon Medical Board

[18] House of Lords Report 86-II (Session 2004-05), Page 257

by OHA, it is reported to the Oregon Medical Board for further investigation[19]*"*.

So, what regulatory role is performed by the Oregon Medical Board? The Mackay Committee was told by representatives of the Board that "*the Board does not go out specifically to monitor any particular issue with physicians. We react only to complaints received*". This was spelled out by the then Medical Director:

> *"The problem we have is if we do not get the complaint we do not investigate it. There may be instances in which there are problems, but if they are not brought to our attention there is no way for us to investigate them. In any area of medical practice, we do not go out and affirmatively go looking for trouble, so to speak"*[20].

For a medical regulatory body this is not an unreasonable stance. But it leaves unanswered the question: who is auditing the quality of the assessment process? The post-event scrutiny that exists is essentially reactive - to apparent irregularities in reporting or to complaints - and is based on a tick-in-the-box procedure. The claim that there has been no abuse of the law may possibly be true, but the evidence to support it is not there.

Waiting Period

As noted above, the DWDA requires a minimum of 15 days to elapse between the two requests for PAS and at least 48 hours to elapse between the submission of a written request and the writing of a prescription for lethal drugs. However, the OHA's website states that *"starting January 1 2020, patients are exempt from any waiting period that exceeds their life expectancy"* and that the 15-day rule does not apply to patients expected to die within that period. It states also that *"patients with less than 48*

---

[19] Oregon Health Authority, Death with Dignity Act, Frequently Asked Questions

[20] House of Lords Report 86-II (Session 2004-05), Page 323

hours to live are exempt from the 48-hour waiting period between the patient's written request and the writing of the DWDA prescription". In such cases *"the Attending Physician must file a medically confirmed certificate of the imminence of the patient's death"*[21].

Most people would agree that for a decision of such gravity a suitable cooling-off period is sensible, though some might wonder whether two weeks provides adequate time for reflection and the forming of a settled wish to die. Be that as it may, to remove the waiting period altogether for people whose deaths are thought to be 'imminent' raises the further question of why it is thought necessary or appropriate to provide people who are very close to or in some cases at the point of death with the means to take their own lives.

Enrolled in Hospice

Some 90 per cent of those who have died in Oregon by physician-assisted suicide since 1997 were recorded as having been enrolled in hospice care. It is important to know what this means. It means that the people concerned were enrolled in hospice programmes. For the greater part this means, not that they were being cared for in hospices, but that they were living at home and being visited by doctors or nurses with a knowledge of palliative care. There is, of course, nothing unusual about hospice-at-home programmes: they exist in the UK alongside the nationwide network of in-patient and day hospices that we have. In Oregon, however, hospice-at-home is the predominant feature of hospice care.

There seems to be general agreement that palliative care has improved in Oregon in recent years. Whether there is a connection between improved palliative care and legalised physician-assisted

---

[21] Oregon Health Authority, Death with Dignity Act, Frequently Asked Questions

suicide is impossible to say. Palliative care has improved in most countries in recent years as a result of advances in medical science and greater focus on health care. According to an Oregon-based researcher, who gave evidence to the Mackay Committee, enactment of the DWDA in the 1990s "*in some ways was a vote of no confidence about some aspects of end of life care in Oregon*"[22].

Palliative medicine in Oregon has only recently achieved the status of a recognised medical specialism. In Britain, by contrast, it has been a recognised clinical speciality, such as (for example) oncology or paediatrics, for over 30 years and there are demanding and mandatory four-year training programmes for those who wish to specialise and reach consultant status.

The Mackay Committee was told when visiting Oregon in 2004 that to qualify for free health care a terminally-ill patient must gain access to a hospice programme, which itself depended on the patient having a prognosis of six months or less of life remaining - ie the same criterion as for physician-assisted suicide. Moreover, the committee was told, entering a hospice programme involved waiving the right to curative treatment. As one witness put it:

> "*It pretty much is a one-way ticket opting out into hospice. The hospice teams are paid governmentally for treatments that are comfort-only. You would not come back to hospital for a CT scan because it would not be paid for*".

The witness added that nearly all patients entering hospice programmes completed a POLST (Physician Order for Life Sustaining Treatment) declaration, "*where they say that they would want comfort measures only, do not resuscitate, no antibiotics except for comfort, probably no artificial hydration or nutrition*"[23].

---

[22] House of Lords Report 86-II (Session 2004-05), Page 281

[23] House of Lords Report (Session 200405) 86-I, Paragraph 157

It is important to be clear on this point as the terms hospice and hospice care do not have exactly the same meaning in Oregon as they have in Britain.

Overall Assessment

It is difficult to deliver a verdict on the working of Oregon's physician-assisted suicide law because there is a paucity of reliable information available as to how requests under the DWDA are being handled in practice. There are plentiful data on how many people have died under its terms, how old they were, what illnesses they had been suffering from and so on. What is needed is information on how the doctors who agree to consider such requests are going about the business of deciding whether the requests before them meet the requirements of the law - for instance, whether they are digging deeper into those requests or simply taking them at face value or whether they are talking to relatives or others who know the applicants well or are contenting themselves with consulting room discussions.

The available data provide a few glimpses of what is happening behind the scenes, not all of which are reassuring. It is clear, for example, that some (perhaps many) people are being assessed for assisted suicide by doctors to whom they have been introduced specifically for the purpose and who can have no first-hand knowledge of them as patients and that some doctors are writing numerous prescriptions for lethal drugs. It is also clear that some of those for whom lethal drugs are prescribed are living significantly beyond the timeframe of terminal illness specified in the law before either ingesting those drugs or dying of natural causes. It is a matter for rejoicing that they are living longer than expected and have apparently not felt the need to take their own lives. But it also highlights the difficulty of making accurate prognoses in cases of terminal illness at ranges such as six months and it raises the question whether there are recipients of lethal drugs who are taking such prognoses at face value and ending their lives prematurely in the belief that they will soon be dead, when in fact they could have months or possibly years of life ahead of them. There is also the concern that few prescribing doctors are present when the lethal drugs they have supplied are ingested, so there is no way of knowing whether the recipients continue to have capacity or have come to feel under pressure of one kind or another to end their lives.

There is also the matter of the rising death rate. It is arguable that the uptake of a new law is bound to rise in its early years. But it is now 22 years since the DWDA came into force and there is no sign of the rising trend in deaths from physician-assisted suicide abating.

The Netherlands[24]

In 2001 The Netherlands passed a law[25] creating an exception to the Criminal Code. Under the Code ending another person's life or assisting a suicide was, and remains today, a criminal offence. The 2001 Act created an exception whereby the Code would not apply if a physician had terminated the life, or assisted the suicide, of a patient on request and if certain 'due care' criteria had been observed.

The 2001 Act formalised what had been a growing practice in The Netherlands over the previous 20 years, during which doctors who had administered voluntary euthanasia or assisted a patient's suicide had been able to invoke a 'defence of necessity' - meaning that they had been able to argue as a defence that ending, or helping to end, the patient's life had been necessary to relieve that patient's suffering.

---

[24] In relation to this section, see also ‘Death on Demand? An Analysis of Physician-Administered Euthanasia in The Netherlands’, by the author and published in the British Medical Bulletin 12 February 2018

[25] Termination of Life on Request and Assisted Suicide (Review Procedures) Act

The Law

Article 2 is the central feature of the 2001 Act. It sets out the 'due care' criteria the observance of which renders an act of voluntary euthanasia or assisted suicide immune from prosecution. It states that the physician must be satisfied that the patient's request is "*voluntary and well-considered*" and that the patient's suffering is "*lasting and unbearable*" with no prospect of improvement. The physician must inform the patient about his or her medical situation and prognosis and consult at least one other, independent doctor and be satisfied, with the patient, that no other reasonable solution to the patient's situation exists. If the physician considers these conditions to have been met, he or she may administer voluntary euthanasia to the patient or assist his or her suicide by supplying a lethal dosage of drugs.

The 2001 Act does not specifically require that the requesting patient should have mental capacity: the presence of capacity is seen an element of a well-considered request. Nor does it require that the patient should have been diagnosed as having a terminal illness. The two principal criteria are a voluntary and well-considered request and lasting and unbearable suffering.

The Act charged regional euthanasia review committees with examining notifications of voluntary euthanasia or assisted suicide submitted by Dutch doctors and adjudicating on whether the requirements of 'due care' had been observed. There are five such regional committees and the 2001 Act requires them collectively to issue annual reports describing their findings.

The Reports

The committees (referred to hereinafter by their Dutch acronym RTEs) have presented a consolidated report for each calendar year from 2002 onwards. These show the number of notifications of PAE and PAS received by them and address issues which have arisen during the year in considering them. To illustrate the latter some anonymised case histories are summarised.

The graph on Page 95 shows the number of cases notified to the RTEs in each year from 2002 to 2019. The five years immediately following the passing of the Act saw a more or less level trend in the numbers of reported cases and it was claimed by some that the warnings of opponents of legalisation had been shown to be groundless. After 2006, however, the annual numbers began to rise. In 2006 there were 1,923 deaths notified to the RTEs as having resulted from PAE or PAS: by 2019 that number had risen to 6,361. This, according to the RTE report on 2019, represented 4.2 per cent of all deaths in The Netherlands. To put it another way, in 2019 one death in every twenty-five in The Netherlands was the result of legalised euthanasia or assisted suicide.

96 per cent of deaths in 2019 were the result of PAE. This predominance of PAE over PAS where both are legally available is not a specifically Dutch phenomenon. Initial reports on the outturn of Canada's 2016 'Medical Assistance in Dying' law indicate a similar pattern.

The RTE report on 2019 states that 4,100 of the 6,361 notified cases in that year were of people who had been diagnosed with incurable cancer. Other conditions included nervous system disorders (408), cardiovascular disease (251) and lung disease (187). Also included in the total were deaths of people with dementia and of others who had been diagnosed with psychiatric conditions. The numbers of deaths of people with psychiatric illness have been on the rise in recent years. In 2011 there were 13 reported cases of euthanasia involving people with psychiatric conditions: by 2019 this had risen to 68. Over the same period the number of people receiving euthanasia or assisted suicide for dementia rose from 49 to 162. In 2019 the RTEs were notified of 172 deaths where those concerned had been suffering from what the report calls an 'accumulation of old-age disorders'. These included

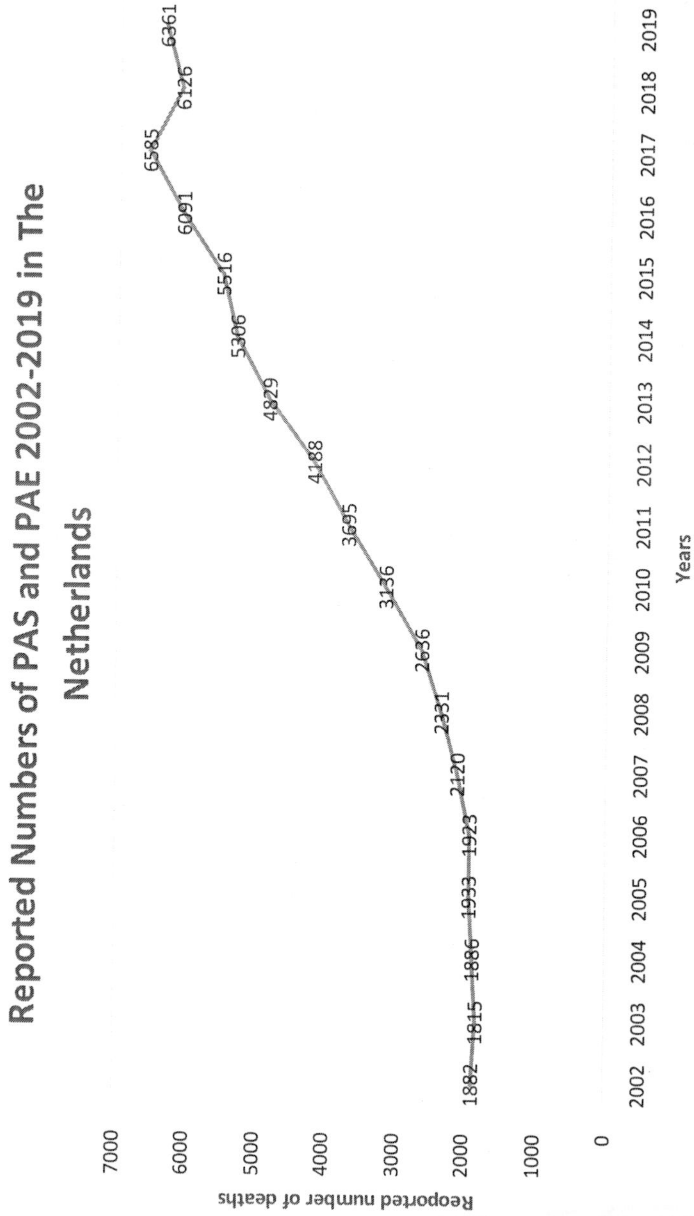
Reported Numbers of PAS and PAE 2002-2019 in The Netherlands
Reported number of deaths
0
1000
2000
3000
4000
5000
6000
7000
1882
1815
1886
1933
1923
2120
2331
2636
3136
3695
4188
4829
5306
5516
6091
6585
6126
6361
2002
2003
2004
2005
2006
2007
2008
2009
2010
2011
2012
2013
2014
2015
2016
2017
2018
2019
Years

sight and hearing disorders, osteoporosis, osteoarthritis, balance problems and cognitive decline. The RTEs ruled that only four (less than 0.01 per cent) of the 6,361 reported cases did not comply with the law.

SCEN

In most cases doctors who consider requests for euthanasia or assisted suicide turn to a group called SCEN (Support and Consultation for Euthanasia in The Netherlands) for the second medical opinion required by the law. SCEN consists of a network of doctors who have been trained to serve as independent consulting physicians and to support the doctors making the decisions. The Mackay Committee was told by a Dutch SCEN physician that *"because of our training, but also because of our experience and the countrywide availability of SCEN physicians, this guarantees a uniform and independent view and…control of the procedure"*. He added that *"after we have carried out our consultation, we give the physician a written report in which we state whether or not the procedure has been completed"*. The committee was also told that, if euthanasia is performed, the SCEN report is sent to the appropriate review committee *"which will give the final judgement"*[26].

Issues

Numbers

The RTE reports tell us how many cases of PAE and PAS have been notified to the committees in each year. But do their figures tell the whole story? Since 1990 quinquennial research studies into end-of-life decision-making have been carried out in The Netherlands. These studies are based on random samples, taken from the central death registry of Statistics Netherlands, of persons whose deaths were registered in the period between

---

[26] House of Lords Report 86-II (Session 2004–05), Page 481

August and November of the years under examination and on anonymous responses from the doctors concerned as to whether an end-of-life decision was involved and, if so, what was its nature. For example, did it comprise withdrawal of life-sustaining treatment? or intensified alleviation of symptoms with a concomitant but unintended risk of hastened death? Or was death caused by PAE or PAS?

The studies commenced prior to legalisation. They indicated a rising reporting rate of euthanasia during the 1990s which, at the time when the 2001 Act was passed, was estimated to have reached 54 per cent. By 2005 it was considered that the reporting rate had reached around 80 per cent and it is generally thought to have remained more or less stable at that level since then. The most recent quinquennial study at the time of writing was concerned with the year 2015.

Against this background it is interesting to compare the numbers of cases notified annually to the RTEs with the estimated numbers of deaths from PAE and PAS based on the studies. According to Statistics Netherlands, in 2015 there were an estimated 6,822 deaths from PAE or PAS, whereas the RTEs reported that 5,516 cases had been notified to them in that year. This conflict of data is not a single-year phenomenon. In 2010 Statistics Netherlands had calculated that there had been 4,051 cases of PAE or PAS in that year, whereas the RTEs had reported that 3,136 cases had been notified to them.

If the data emerging from the quinquennial studies are correct, this raises the question: why are these additional numbers of deaths not being reported by the doctors concerned to the RTEs? According to the research report on 2010, "*in the unreported cases the drugs used were hardly ever neuromuscular relaxants*" - the drugs most commonly used in euthanasia. This might suggest that these excess deaths were the result of intensified alleviation of symptoms through administration of opioids rather than drugs administered with the aim of bringing about death. On the other hand, the report states that these cases were classified as euthanasia only when the physicians concerned affirmed that there was an intention to end the patient's life.

It is difficult to know what to make of this. There does seem, however, to be a grey area as regards the actual incidence of euthanasia in The Netherlands and that the RTEs' annual reports might not tell the whole story.

Scrutiny

As noted above, the 2001 Act placed responsibility with the RTEs for assessing reports of euthanasia and assisted suicide and deciding whether the requirements of the law had been observed. The committees are, however, doing more than deciding whether or not the law has been broken. They are also determining the precise boundaries of the law by ruling on whether, and in what circumstances, certain acts or situations fall within the law's 'due care' criteria. The committees were clear about this role from the outset. In their first annual report following legalisation, they stated that "*the committees do have some latitude interpreting the due care criteria*" and that "*the question of how the criteria are to be applied in specific cases is left up to them*"[27].

This role is perhaps inevitable given the nature of the criteria as laid down in the Act. Some of these are fairly clear-cut - for example, that there should have been an independent second-opinion and that the patient should have been informed of his or her condition and prognosis. But other, important, criteria - such as the need for a request to be voluntary and well-considered or for the patient's suffering to be lasting and unbearable and with no prospect of improvement - offer considerable scope for subjective judgement. Given the open nature of the criteria laid down in the

---

[27] Regional Euthanasia Review Committees Report 2002

Act, the committees seem to have found themselves obliged, in reaching their judgements in individual cases, to formulate their own guidelines for assessing whether acts of euthanasia or assisted suicide comply with the law. In effect, therefore, the committees are developing the law as well as deciding who has and who has not broken it.

In 2015 the RTEs published a Code of Practice to outline "*the issues and considerations that the committees regard as relevant in connection with the statutory due care criteria for euthanasia*'[28]. The Code draws a distinction between individual 'due care' criteria and the levels of scrutiny given to them. It states that, in regard to some of the criteria (whether the deceased patient had been informed of his or her situation and prognosis, whether another independent physician had been consulted and whether the patient's life had been terminated with due medical care), "*it must be clear that the physician complied with the due care criteria*". However, in regard to others (whether the request was voluntary and well-considered, whether the patient's suffering was unbearable and had no prospect of improvement and there was no reasonable alternative to euthanasia), the physician must be able to "*plausibly argue that, given the circumstances of the case, he was reasonably able to conclude*" that these tests had been met[29]. The committees' 2016 report suggests that this process "*would be described by Dutch lawyers as 'limited review' or a test of reasonableness*"[30]

According to the committees' 2016 report, this means that "*the RTEs do not carry out a full review of compliance with the due care criteria and therefore do not re-examine the same issues as the*

---

[28] Regional Euthanasia Review Committees Code of Practice, The Hague, April 2015, Page 5

[29] Regional Euthanasia Review Committees Code of Practice, The Hague, April 2015, Page 5

[30] RTEs Annual Report for 2016

physician who made the original decision. The RTEs cannot do this, as the patient is no longer alive: these are the issues that the independent physician focuses on"[31]. This is an important admission. The committees are acknowledging that in respect of these key criteria they are not examining whether the notifying doctor's action was correct, that they are in effect sub-contracting that function to the 'second opinion' doctor and that their role in respect of these key criteria is to assess whether, based on the information given to them and the plausibility of the doctor's arguments, the decision to provide PAS or PAE seemed reasonable.

A study published in 2017[32] of cases where the RTEs had ruled that the 'due care' criteria had not been met observed that "*the majority of cases did not meet the due care criteria for procedural or technical reasons*" and that "*even when the substantive criteria were at issue, the RTEs' focus was generally not on whether the physician had made a 'correct' judgement but on whether the physician followed a thorough process (ie whether physicians should have consulted specialists or evaluated the patient further), but not on whether the patient should have received Euthanasia or Assisted Suicide*" (EAS). The study concluded:

> "*Evaluating EAS requests requires complicated judgements in implementing criteria that are intentionally open-ended, evolving and fraught with acknowledged interpretive difficulties. Our review suggests that the Dutch review system's primary mode of handling this difficulty is a trust-based system that focuses on the procedural thoroughness and professionalism of physicians*"

The 'limited review' approach could be seen as a serious weakness in the Dutch system. Decisions by doctors to grant PAE or PAS may well follow the processes correctly but may nonetheless be

---

[31] RTEs Annual Report for 2016

[32] Miller, DG, Kim, SYH, Euthanasia and assisted suicide not meeting due care criteria in the Netherlands: a qualitative review of review committee judgements, BMJ 2017:7:bmjopen.bmj.com/content/7/10/e017628

misguided. Ensuring that a person making such a request has been informed of his or her diagnosis and prognosis and that a second opinion has been sought are relatively straightforward matters. But assessing whether a request is voluntary and well-considered and involves unbearable suffering with no reasonable alternative to euthanasia calls for the exercise of difficult judgements. An effective system of case review must arguably examine those judgements as well as the processes that led up to them.

There is another consideration to be borne in mind in assessing the robustness of the RTEs' scrutiny of PAE and PAS deaths. All audit activity, if it is to be effective, requires a sceptical and detached mindset. In financial or business audit or other areas of activity where there is consensus over the underlying aims and values, finding auditors with these characteristics does not present a serious problem. Euthanasia, on the other hand, is a controversial and divisive social issue in which there are strongly-held views on both sides of the political debate. This raises the question: how are impartial and objective scrutineers to be found who are sufficiently unencumbered by 'baggage' (on both sides of the debate) to review reported acts of PAE or PAS dispassionately and with an appropriate degree of challenge?

The same issue arises in relation to the SCEN network. While the existence of a nationwide network of second-opinion doctors who are trained and experienced in the application of the 2001 Act has some obvious advantages in terms of availability and consistency, it could be argued that it places the process in the hands of doctors who are, by reason of their membership of the network, supportive of legalised euthanasia.

Doctor-Patient Relationships

When the Mackay Committee visited The Netherlands in 2004, just three years following legalisation, it was told by a member of the euthanasia review committee covering The Hague:

"There is an absolute condition that it [euthanasia] can only be done by the treating physician. It cannot be any other physician. We do not want to advertise euthanasia tourism. What we insist on is that it only takes place within a meaningful medical relationship. That is an absolute condition"[33].

This highlights what has been until recently a distinctive feature of euthanasia in The Netherlands. PAE or PAS has generally been provided by GPs to patients on their lists rather than by referral doctors who step in when a patient's regular doctor declines to participate or to agree to a request.

However, the RTEs’ 2012 report stated that 32 notifications of PAE/PAS had been received in that year from doctors who were connected with a body known as the Levenseinde Klinik (End of Life Clinic). This body, since re-named as the Euthanasia Expertise Centre (EE), considers requests that have been rejected or referred by patients' regular doctors. By the time of the 2016 report the number of EE-associated deaths from euthanasia had risen to 487: by 2018 it had reached 726. The RTEs’ report on 2019 states that 904 of the cases notified to them had involved the EE. This represents one in seven of all cases notified and a 25 per cent increase on the year before.

Doctors who do not perform euthanasia for reasons of principle or who will only perform euthanasia if the patient has a terminal condition or who consider a request over-complex may refer patients to the EE. Such a referral may also be initiated by the patient or his or her family. The RTEs’ report on 2018 stated that 65 per cent of notified cases of PAE or PAS of patients with a psychiatric disorder came from EE physicians, as did over 40 per cent of those involving a form of dementia and just under 40 per cent of cases where there had been multiple geriatric syndromes.

---

[33] House of Lords Report 86-II (Session 2004-05), Page 436

It would appear therefore that a long-term doctor-patient relationship as a basis for euthanasia is no longer the absolute condition that it was considered to be when the law was changed.

Overall Assessment

There are some features of the Dutch 2001 law that are commendable. The very title of the law - Termination of Life on Request and Assisted Suicide Act - is admirably clear and comes as a refreshing change from the evasive and euphemistic phraseology and linguistic contortions – such as Death with Dignity, End of Life Options, Medical Assistance in Dying - which have characterised similar ending-life laws in other jurisdictions and which can be seen in the use by campaigners in Britain of the term 'assisted dying'.

Another positive feature of the Dutch law is its provision for post-event scrutiny of acts of PAE and PAS. Effective scrutiny is needed both to deter malpractice and laxity and to provide transparency. The problem is that the system of scrutiny adopted appears to lack sufficient rigour to meet these requirements. A 'pass rate' in excess of 99.5 per cent is not easy to credit and the methodology of review raises questions as to whether the RTEs are examining the judgements that doctors are making as well as the processes they are following.

A major difference of the Dutch 2001 Act from Oregon's DWDA is that it allows PAE as well as PAS. PAE accounts for more than 95 per cent of deaths under the Act and results in a much higher overall death rate. Why should this be so? Perhaps, with its involvement of doctors in administering lethal drugs rather than just supplying them to qualifying patients, it is because it places the patient in the position of passive recipient rather than active participant. Perhaps also the direct involvement of doctors leads to PAE being perceived or misperceived by patients as having attributes of medical care. Whatever the reasons, it is indisputable that, where PAE is legalised alongside PAS, it has the effect of driving out the latter and driving up the numbers of hastened deaths dramatically. A law in England and Wales along the lines of the Dutch 2001 Act would, on current death rates, result in some 23,000 deaths a year.

The incremental spread of PAE and PAS in The Netherlands into new types of medical condition, such as psychiatric disorders, dementia and multiple geriatric ailments, can raise eyebrows but should not surprise us. The 2001 Act was framed in fairly broad terms and is open to elastic interpretation. Laws in other jurisdictions, such as Oregon, set what might appear to be more restrictive parameters such as terminal illness and a prognosis of six months or less of life remaining. But they beg the question: if the relief of suffering is to be the touchstone for ending or providing the means for ending people's lives, where is the logic in providing such help to people who are expected to die shortly of natural causes but withholding it from others with chronic conditions who may have years of discomfort ahead of them?

One insider who has expressed serious doubts about the 2001 Act is Dr Theo Boer, a professional ethicist who was a member of one of the RTEs and in that capacity reviewed over 4,000 cases. In July 2014 Dr Boer expressed his concerns in the British press:

> "*For the first five years after the law became effective, such physician-induced deaths remained level - and even fell in some years. In 2007 I wrote that 'there doesn't need to be a slippery slope when it comes to euthanasia. A good euthanasia law, in combination with the euthanasia review procedure, provides the warrants for a stable and relatively low number of euthanasias'. Most of my colleagues drew the same conclusion. But we were wrong - terribly wrong, in fact. In hindsight, the stabilisation in the numbers was just a temporary pause. Beginning in 2008 the*

> *numbers of these deaths show a 15% increase annually, year after year"*[34].

Dr Boer drew attention to the sharp rise in the numbers of people with psychiatric conditions who were receiving euthanasia or assisted suicide. He did not believe this was the end of the road. The campaigners, he wrote, "*will not rest until a lethal pill is made available to anyone over 70 years who wishes to die*".

Referring to the pressures on doctors, from both patients and their relatives, Dr Boer said that "*not even the review committees, despite hard and conscientious work, have been able to halt these developments.* He concluded:

> *"I used to be a supporter of the Dutch law. But now, with twelve years experience, I take a very different view. At the very least, wait for an honest and intellectually satisfying analysis of the reasons behind the explosive increase in the numbers. Is it because the law should have had better safeguards? Or is it because the mere existence of such a law is an invitation to see assisted suicide and euthanasia as a normality instead of a last resort? Before those questions are answered, don't go there. Once the genie is out of the bottle, it is not likely to ever go back in again".*

Canada

Introduction

Canada has a larger population than any of the jurisdictions that have gone down the road of legalising PAS or PAE – some 37 million compared with around 17 million for The Netherlands and 4 million for Oregon.

However, for a number of reasons there are difficulties in presenting an objective account of Canada's experience. Whereas in Oregon and The Netherlands legalisation led immediately to the

---

[34] Daily Mail, 10 July 2014

publication of official annual reports on the take-up and characteristics of PAS and PAE, the Canadian Government's output to date has been limited to the publication of four 'interim' reports covering the period up to October 2018 and a recent statement of overall annual numbers covering the period 2016 to 2019. In a document published in January 2020 the Federal Government announced that *"on November 1 2018 a new federal monitoring regime, including a more robust data collection system, came into effect"* and that *"the federal government will begin annual public reporting on MAiD, using information collected under this new regime, starting in the Spring of 2020"*[35]. It now seems that the first such report will not appear before the end of summer 2020[36].

There are also two laws on this subject in Canada. In December 2015 the Province of Quebec passed an 'Act Respecting End of Life Care', one section of which permits 'medical aid in dying'. Six months later, in June 2016, the Federal Government enacted its 'Medical Assistance in Dying' (MAiD) law for Canada's other Provinces and Territories. While these two pieces of legislation are broadly similar, on some important points they differ – for example, Quebec's law permits only physician-administered euthanasia, whereas the federal 2016 MAiD law permits both PAE and physician-assisted suicide.

Another problem in writing about Canada at this time is that legislation permitting the supply or administration of lethal drugs resembles a building still under construction. Quebec has recently removed from its 2015 law the requirement that an applicant's death must be 'reasonably foreseeable' before euthanasia may be administered; and the Federal Government has tabled a similar amendment to its own MAiD law. There is also discussion taking place as to whether other changes (for example, regarding people

---

[35] 'Medical assistance in dying', document published by the Government of Canada, 13 January 2020.

[36] Correspondence between the author and Health Canada

who are mentally ill) should be made. Inevitably, therefore, what is said in this section is vulnerable to being overtaken by events.

Yet another complication is that implementation of the federal 2016 MAiD law has been devolved to Provinces and Territories. A document published by the Government of Canada in January 2020 stated that *"policies and procedures for medical assistance in dying may vary among provinces and territories"*[37]. It gives, as an example, Quebec's legalisation of PAE but not of PAS. While it is possible therefore to provide a broadly-based picture of the situation in Canada, there may be variations in practice.

Against this background the following paragraphs attempt to describe Canada's legislation in fairly broad terms, to give what information is available on its outturn to date and to draw attention to known developments.

Requirements of the Law

The federal 2016 Medical Assistance in Dying (MAiD) legislation was enacted in response to a Judgment of the Supreme Court of Canada that the existing law in this area was in conflict with the Canadian Charter of Rights and Freedoms. The Court required the Government to change the law by a specified date and, in response, the Government enacted its MAiD legislation in June 2016.

As enacted in 2016, Canada's MAiD law permitted lethal drugs to be supplied or administered by a doctor or (in Provinces where allowed) a nurse practitioner subject to certain conditions. These were that the person requesting MAiD must be 18 years of age or over, have a *'grievous and irremediable medical condition'*, be free from external pressure and give informed consent. In the law as enacted in 2016 a grievous and irremediable medical condition was defined as a condition where a person had *"a serious and*

[37] Medical Assistance in Dying, Government of Canada, 13 January 2020

incurable illness, disease or disability" and was *"in an advanced state of irreversible decline in capability".* That condition should cause the person *"enduring physical or psychological suffering that is intolerable to them and that cannot be relieved under conditions that they consider acceptable",* and *"their natural death has become reasonably foreseeable*[38]*".*

So far as process was concerned, a doctor or nurse practitioner considering a request for MAiD must receive a written request which has been signed by two independent witnesses, must ensure that the applicant meets all the above criteria and must have his or her judgement confirmed by another, independent, doctor or nurse practitioner. Where a decision to provide MAiD was made, the 2016 law required an applicant to wait at least ten days before PAS or PAE was performed. In the words of the Government of Canada, *"If you do decide to proceed after the 10 days, your practitioner can have confidence in your true desire to receive the service"*[39]. This period of reflection would not apply if the patient's death or loss of decision-making capacity were considered to be fast approaching.

MAiD does not seem to have included any arrangements for post-event scrutiny of deaths from PAS or PAE. The legislation requires the Minister of Health to *"make regulations that he or she considers necessary...respecting the provision and collection, for the purpose of monitoring medical assistance in dying, of information relating to requests for, and the provision of, medical assistance in dying*[40]*".* On 28 July 2018 the Government of Canada published Regulations for the Monitoring of Medical Assistance in Dying. These, among other things, empower the Minister of Health *"for the purpose of monitoring medical assistance in dying, to collect personal information relating to written requests for, and*

---

[38] Bill C-14 (Medical Assistance in Dying), Section 241(2)

[39] Medical Assistance in Dying, Government of Canada, 13 January 2020

[40] Bill C-14 (Medical Assistance in Dying), Section 241.31(3)

the provision of, medical assistance in dying from a provincial or territorial government or any of its institutions"[41]. The regulations also state that "*the Minister of Health must cause to be published, at least once a year, on the website of the Government of Canada a report that is based on information that the Minister obtained under these Regulations"*[42].

However, though the regulations require that information be provided on procedural requirements (for example, which criteria for MAiD had been assessed and what information had been provided to patients), they do not seem to involve qualitative review of the process of assessment. Indeed, a Regulatory Impact Analysis Statement published with the regulations draws a distinction between the gathering of data for monitoring purposes and a case review system. It states:

> *"The monitoring regime is aimed at gathering and analyzing data about medical assistance in dying from a societal perspective. It is fundamentally distinct from a process that seeks to assess individual medical or nurse practitioners' compliance with the Criminal Code exemptions. Investigating instances of non-compliance with the eligibility criteria and procedural safeguards set out in the Criminal Code falls outside the scope of the federal monitoring regime and is under the purview of local law enforcement"*[43].

Evolution

A document published by the Government of Canada in March 2020 includes a paragraph headed 'Evolution of MAID in Canada'. Under this heading it is stated that "*during the development and implementation of MAID (Bill C-14), many Canadians voiced their*

---

[41] Regulations for the Monitoring of Medical Assistance in Dying, July 2018, Section 12(1)

[42] Regulations for the Monitoring of Medical Assistance in Dying, July 2018, Section 13(1)

[43] Regulations for the Monitoring of Medical Assistance in Dying, July 2018, Regulatory Impact Analysis Statement

support for broader access to MAID" and that the Government *"committed to study a wider variety of medical circumstances where a person may want to access MAID"*. The document goes on to say that the Government asked the Council of Canadian Academies to study three issues – requests for MAiD from 'mature minors', advance requests for MAiD and *"requests for people where mental illness is the only reason for requesting MAID"*[44] – it is interesting that the document talks of requests 'for' rather than requests 'by' people with mental illness.

Only four years after the enactment of MAiD its parameters are being changed. On 24 February 2020 the Government introduced a bill to amend the 2016 law's provisions. This followed a ruling in September 2019 by the Superior Court of Quebec that the requirement in MAiD that death should be "*reasonably foreseeable*" and in the Province's own legislation that a patient should be "*at the end of life*" was unconstitutional. These requirements ceased to be applicable in the Province of Quebec as of 12 March 2020.

According to a Government of Canada document, "*the proposed changes follow extensive consultations with Canadians, experts, practitioners, stakeholders, Indigenous groups, provinces and territories"*[45]. The document stated that there was to be "*a two-track approach to procedural safeguards based on whether or not a person's natural death is reasonably foreseeable"*. "*Existing safeguards"*, it stated, *"will be maintained and eased for persons whose death is reasonably foreseeable. New and strengthened safeguards would be applied to eligible persons whose death is not reasonably foreseeable"*.

The main relaxations in MAiD may be summarised as follows:

---

44 Government of Canada, Medical Assistance in Dying, January and February 2020 Consultations

45 Government of Canada, Proposed changes to Canada's medical assistance in dying legislation, 26 February 2020

- Removal of the requirement that death should be 'reasonably foreseeable';
- Requirement for only one independent witness to a request for MAiD;
- A paid personal or health care worker may be an independent witness;
- Removal of the requirement that there should be a 10-day period for reflection;
- Waiver of the requirement for final consent to MAiD before it is provided where death is reasonably foreseeable and consent has been given in advance.

Other changes to the 2016 legislation are:

- A requirement that one of the two practitioners who assess eligibility must have expertise in the medical condition that is causing the person's suffering;
- A mental illness is not to be regarded as a 'serious and incurable illness, disease or disability'
- Introduction of a minimum period of 90 days for consideration of a request where death is not reasonably foreseeable. This period can, however, be reduced if loss of capacity is considered to be imminent and assessments are complete;
- A requirement that an applicant for MAiD must be informed of counselling, mental health support, disability support, community services and palliative care and be offered consultation with relevant professionals, as available and applicable;

Data

According to the Government of Canada[46], there were 13,712 deaths resulting from MAiD and Quebec's Act Respecting End of

---

[46] Government of Canada, An Act to Amend the Criminal Code (medical assistance in dying), Technical Briefing 24 February 2020

Life Care in the four years from 2016 to 2019 – though the figure for 2019 was said to be 'still under revision'. The number of deaths in 2019 (5,444) was said to represent 1.89 per cent of all deaths in Canada in that year. The four interim reports, covering the period from June 2016 to October 2018, show that deaths from MAiD were overwhelmingly the result of PAE rather than PAS. The interim reports recorded only six cases of PAS. This reflects, as we have seen earlier in this chapter, the experience of The Netherlands that, where both PAS and PAE are on offer, the latter is the near-invariable practice and the numbers of deaths are substantial.

Freedom of Conscience

The preamble to the MAiD legislation states that "*everyone has freedom of conscience and religion under Section 2 of the Canadian Charter of Rights and Freedoms*", that "*nothing in this Act affects the guarantee of freedom of conscience and religion*" and that "*the Government of Canada has committed to…respect the personal convictions of health care providers*". Doctors and nurse practitioners are not, therefore, obliged by the law to process requests for MAiD. However, how these principles are put into effect has been delegated to Provinces and Territories, some of whom require practitioners who decline to process a request for MAiD to refer the patient to another practitioner who is willing to do so.

Comment

At this stage it would be premature to offer a verdict on Canada's MAiD legislation. Any conclusions drawn must be provisional given the shifting nature of the MAiD legislation and the paucity, at the time of writing, of official data on the law's outturn.

As noted above, enactment of MAiD derived from a Canadian Supreme Court Judgment. In the words of the Government of

Canada, *"the Supreme Court gave the government until June 6 2016 to create a new law"*[47]. Those words are telling. Though the Federal Parliament had discretion over what the new law should be, it had no choice but to change the law and to do so by a Court-prescribed deadline. And, even when the new law has come into effect, it appears to be subject to amendment in response to further Court Judgments.

In Britain Parliament is supreme in the legislative process. The courts may make Judgments as to whether a law is in need of change, and there have been a number of attempts by campaigners for 'assisted dying' to secure such Judgments. But, if the Supreme Court were ever to declare that the current law in this area was in need of change, it would be for Parliament to decide whether the law should be changed. The position was made clear in May 2020 by the Lord Chancellor and Secretary of State for Justice, Robert Buckland QC MP, when he stated that any change in the law on 'assisted dying' was a matter for Parliament.

Against this background and given the changes which are being made to MAiD when the ink is barely dry on the statute it is fair to ask whether the preparation of the law against a court-imposed deadline was unduly rushed. The subject with which MAiD deals is complex and controversial and the consequences of error are grave. MAiD is beginning to look less like a piece of considered legislation and more like a starting point.

What are we to make of the most recent amendments? Even before withdrawal of the requirement that death should be reasonably foreseeable the Government of Canada had stated that *"you do **not** need to have a fatal or terminal condition to be eligible for medical assistance in dying*[48]*"*. Withdrawal of the requirement that death should be reasonably foreseeable leaves little doubt that, whatever its title may suggest, MAiD is about providing help

[47] Medical Assistance in Dying, Government of Canada, 13 January 2020
[48] Medical Assistance in Dying, Government of Canada, 13 January 2020

to end their lives not only to people who are dying but also to others with chronic rather than terminal illnesses.

The requirement that, where death is not reasonably foreseeable, there should be a period of at least 90 days for assessment of a request looks, at first sight, like a step in the right direction. Most people would surely agree that such life-or-death decisions should not be rushed and that both those who make requests for MAiD and those who consider those requests should take the time required for mature reflection and careful and painstaking assessment. However, this new safeguard may be overridden where an assessment is complete in less than 90 days and loss of capacity is thought to be imminent.

The introduction of the 90-day rule has also to be balanced against the removal of the ten-day period of reflection for people whose death is considered to be reasonably foreseeable. This safeguard was already open to objection by reason of the caveat that it did not apply where death or loss of capacity was considered to be imminent. Just why it is regarded as important to end the life of a person who is about to die of natural causes is far from clear. That aside, the removal of the ten-day period of reflection withdraws from persons whose death is reasonably foreseeable – a term which could include people with prognoses of months or more - the protection of a mandatory period of reflection.

The latest changes state that *"for the purposes of MAiD eligibility, a mental illness is* ***not*** *a 'serious and incurable illness, disease or disability"*. While that is helpful as a statement, it has to be asked for how long it will survive as a policy. As noted above, the Government has asked the Council of Canadian Academies to conduct a review of whether requests where a mental disorder is the sole underlying medical condition should qualify for MAiD.

The potential conflict between protecting freedom of conscience of doctors and requiring them to refer requests to other practitioners has been a source of controversy. A recent article in a medical journal referred to tensions in the Province of Ontario over *"regulatory bodies threatening severe punishment for individual healthcare providers who do not initiate "effective" referrals for MAiD[49]"*.

Those with a conscientious objection to providing MAiD may reasonably argue that having to refer a requesting patient to another practitioner who is known to be willing to participate is tantamount to providing MAiD at one remove and, as such, is a violation of conscience. When the Mackay Committee considered Lord Joffe's 2004 Assisted Dying for the Terminally Ill Bill at Westminster, it recommended that any future bill *"should not place on a physician with conscientious objection the duty to refer an applicant for assisted suicide or voluntary euthanasia to another physician without such objection"[50]*. The committee's recommendation, which reflected the view expressed by Parliament's Joint Committee on Human Rights, was accepted at the time by Lord Joffe himself and no proposal requiring doctors with a conscientious objection to make referrals to other practitioners has been included in any subsequent bill.

Many doctors have such conscientious objections, which may stem either from faith-based convictions or from a perceived conflict between administering or prescribing lethal drugs and the ethics of medical practice. It is surely possible to respect those objections without requiring the doctors concerned to find other physicians who are willing to engage in these practices. The Dutch SCEN model (see above) would seem to provide a basis for addressing this issue. A similar arrangement in Canada would enable physicians willing to engage in MAiD to enrol anonymously in a

---

[49] Carpenter, T., Vivas, L. Ethical arguments against coercing provider participation in MAiD (medical assistance in dying) in Ontario, Canada. *BMC Med Ethics* **21,** 46 (2020). https://doi.org/10.1186/s12910-020-00486-2

[50] House of Lords Report 86-I (Session 2004-05), Paragraph 269 (viii)

network of like-minded colleagues. It would be open to an applicant for MAiD whose doctor declines to participate to approach the network for a replacement. According to the article quoted above, a system along these lines is already in existence in the Province of Alberta, where *"a Central Coordination Service (CCS) facilitates referrals for MAiD without requiring clinician participation. This system has a low barrier to access, making it accessible to patients as well as clinicians"*[51].

The Government of Canada has stated (see above) that deaths from MAiD in 2019 represented 1.89 per cent of all deaths in Canada in that year. Its observation that *"in other permissive regimes, assisted deaths account for 0.3% to 4.6% of all deaths* [52] may perhaps be intended to suggest that Canada's experience is within death rates seen in other permissive jurisdictions. If so, it is potentially misleading. At the same stage in the evolution of Dutch euthanasia law the number of deaths reported to have been from PAE and PAS was less than one third of the number reported in The Netherlands in 2019.

Moreover, at that time (2005) the numbers in The Netherlands were relatively stable following legalisation, but shortly afterwards began their climb to where they are now and where reported deaths account for 4.2 per cent of all deaths. Canada's numbers have been rising steeply from the outset – from 1,014 in 2016, to 2,816 in 2017, to 4,438 in 2018 to 5,444 in 2019. The government document describes this rise as *"a consistent and gradual increase"*. This seems a somewhat questionable assessment. It is perhaps noteworthy that, in determining the administrative burden of monitoring MAiD, there was an assumption that

---

[51] Carpenter, T., Vivas, L. Ethical arguments against coercing provider participation in MAiD (medical assistance in dying) in Ontario, Canada. *BMC Med Ethics* **21,** 46 (2020). https://doi.org/10.1186/s12910-020-00486-2

[52] Government of Canada, An Act to Amend the Criminal Code (medical assistance in dying), Technical Briefing 24 February 2020

"Canada would reach a steady state of 2.05% of total deaths attributed to medical assistance in dying". This assumption was *"based on the proportion of deaths resulting from medical assistance in dying in other jurisdictions that permit medical assistance in dying[53]"*. After only four years the estimate of 2.05 per cent of deaths has all but been reached. It is still early days but it does look as though Canada is well embarked on the road to equal if not to surpass the Dutch experience in terms of numbers of deaths.

According to Health Canada[54], *"provinces and territories may establish health-related legislation/policies on MAID as long as they are consistent with the federal MAID legislation. In practice this means that provinces and territories are able to establish policies that are more narrow than the federal law, but not broader. For example, although it is permitted in the federal legislation, Quebec's end-of-life care law does not permit MAID by self-administration and only allows physicians, not nurse practitioners, to assess and provide MAID"*. What this seems to amount to is that the federal MAiD legislation represents a framework within the boundaries of which individual provinces and territories may enact their own laws.

Switzerland

The Law

Switzerland's law in this area is different in nature from others. Switzerland has not passed a law legalising either physician-assisted suicide or physician-administered euthanasia. Under Article 114 of the Swiss Penal Code the killing of a human being, even at the latter's request, is a criminal offence, so voluntary

---

[53] Regulations for the Monitoring of Medical Assistance in Dying, July 2018, Regulatory Impact Analysis Statement

[54] Correspondence with the author

euthanasia is illegal. However, while Article 115 prohibits incitement to and assistance with suicide if the guilty party acts from self-interest, it exempts those who act from non-self-serving motives. Self-interest, the Mackay Committee was told on a visit to the Swiss Federal Ministry of Justice in 2005, includes such situations as where assistance with suicide was given to satisfy the assister's material or emotional needs or to eliminate a family problem or to gain an inheritance or to be rid of a care burden or to eliminate a person whom the assister dislikes. The onus rests on the person giving assistance to demonstrate after the event that his or her assistance was altruistic.

Assisted Suicide and Doctors

Switzerland is different in another respect from those jurisdictions which have assisted suicide laws. Its exemption of assisted suicide from prosecution in certain circumstances was not framed in the context of relieving seriously ill persons from suffering. It is essentially a social libertarian measure dating back to 1942. As the Mackay Committee was told by the Federal Ministry of Justice:

> "*It was not something revolutionary or new and it was not intended to facilitate the killing of hopelessly sick individuals. It did not have anything to do with euthanasia and with right-to-die organisations. This phenomenon has been developing since the eighties*"[55]

Suicide Organisations

Most instances of assistance with suicide in Switzerland are managed by right-to-die organisations, which provide a framework for requests from individuals to be considered, for assistance with suicide to be provided in appropriate cases and for evidence to be provided to the police after an assisted suicide has taken place that the assistance given was within the law. The main such organisation

---

[55] House of Lords Report 86-II (Session 2004-05), Page 607

is Exit, which provides its services solely for Swiss nationals. Another organisation, Dignitas, provides a similar service both for Swiss and non-Swiss nationals.

Over the period from 2002 to 2019 a total of 457[56] Britons ended their lives at the Dignitas assisted suicide facility, an average of about 25 a year. The trend has been uneven but rising: 2016 saw the highest number, when 47 Britons travelled to Dignitas to receive assistance with suicide. This figure represented 0.008 per cent of deaths of UK-based persons in 2016.

Research published in 2014[57] examined the characteristics of over 1,300 assisted suicides managed by Exit and Dignitas between 2003 and 2008. It found that assisted suicide was more likely among women than among men, among people living alone than among those living with others, among those with no religious affiliation than among Protestants or Catholics, among more than less educated people, among those living in urban than others in rural areas and among people of higher socio-economic status. As we have seen, a similar pattern is observable in Oregon. The age range was also similar: two thirds of the cases examined were of elderly people, with the main group within that category being those aged 65-84.

The authors found that "*in older people assisted suicide was more likely in the divorced compared with the married*". Commenting on the higher rate of assisted suicide among people living alone or divorced, the report comments that "*social isolation and loneliness are well-known risk factors for non-assisted suicide*" and that "*our results suggest that they may also play a role in assisted suicide*". Another finding was that "*in younger people, having children was*

---

[56] Statista, Annual Number of Accompanied Suicides to Dignitas in Switzerland from Great Britain from 2002 to 2019

[57] Suicide assisted by right-to-die associations: a population based cohort study, Steck, N et al, International Journal of Epidemiology 2014, 1-9 doi: 10.1093/ije/dyu010

associated with a lower rate". It is of interest that this correlation was not found among older people with children. It raises the question whether having responsibilities for others - or, as some might put it, having something to live for - might perhaps be a restraining factor in decisions to seek assistance with suicide.

In Conclusion

In these four sample jurisdictions (Oregon, The Netherlands, Canada and Switzerland), we see three different approaches to the concept of 'assisted dying'. In Oregon we see a limitation of 'assisted dying' to physician-assisted suicide and an attempt to specify limits to eligibility. The death rate is smaller, though it is rising year by year. Many doctors are unwilling to participate in PAS, with the result that the phenomenon of 'doctor shopping' has grown up, bringing into question the knowledge base on which decisions to provide assisted suicide are taken. The conditions of eligibility for PAS sound fine on paper as general statements but, as we will see in Chapter Seven, they pose some very real difficulties in interpretation. How in practice they are being interpreted is not easy to see in the absence of a post-event system of qualitative scrutiny.

The Netherlands has legalised not only physician-assisted suicide but also physician-administered euthanasia. The 2001 law, moreover, is drafted in fairly open terms which can be interpreted as embracing both physiological and psychological illness and chronic as well as terminal illness. There is a candour about the Dutch law which it is difficult not to respect. There is no attempt to hide what the law really means, and the provision of post-event review arrangements, with their public discussion of problems and case illustrations, betokens an openness which can only be respected.

On the other hand, the continuing and substantial year-on-year rises in deaths from PAS and PAE, especially the latter, and the migration of these practices into mental health, dementia and age-related morbidities is worrying. And, while the concept of post-event audit by the review committees is commendable, its rigour and effectiveness are open to question

It is difficult to know what to make of the situation in Canada. MAiD is only four years old and its parameters have not yet stabilised. The 2016 law looks more like a work in progress than a considered piece of legislation and one cannot help wondering whether its enactment might have been unduly rushed to meet a court-imposed deadline. The outturn to date is also worrying. On the limited official information available annual numbers of deaths are rising rapidly, with PAE even more predominant than in Holland.

In some respects the Swiss legal position is not too far removed from that in England and Wales: assisting suicide is illegal but may not be prosecuted under certain circumstances. Switzerland also appears to have recognised the difficulty of reconciling assisted suicide with the practice of medicine. Doctors are not banned from engaging in such acts: they are in the same position as other citizens in such circumstances. But, insofar as assistance with suicide is allowed in Switzerland, it is not *physician*-assisted suicide but more the province of right-to-die organisations. It is difficult to know what to make of these latter. Concern about their activities was expressed to the Mackay Committee during its visit to Switzerland in 2005[58] and the concept does not seem to have commended itself to campaigners for legal change elsewhere.

It might have been expected that, as evidence mounts regarding the operation of such laws where they have been enacted overseas, a more cautious approach would be adopted to the framing of new legislative proposals. There is, however, little sign of this happening. In England and Wales the parliamentary Private

---

[58] House of Lords Report (Session 2004-05) 86-I, Paragraphs 207-208

Member bills that have been seen in recent years have been close to reproductions of Oregon's DWDA. This failure to take on board the lessons from overseas outturn is one of the most puzzling features of the UK 'assisted dying' debate.

CHAPTER SIX

THE MORAL DIMENSION

ILORA FINLAY AND ROBERT PRESTON

Our morality is the code that governs how we behave

Some say that helping terminally-ill people to end their lives is a compassionate response to their suffering. Others argue that helping people to commit suicide cuts across the natural instinct of humanity to protect life. In this chapter we look at the moral dimension of the 'assisted dying' debate.

Definitions

We need to start by defining our terms. Our morality is the code that governs how we behave. This may have either a transcendental or a secular basis. That is to say, it may rest on a belief that true existence transcends this life (as expressed, for example, in a religious creed) or it may rest on a humanistic view that our life is limited to the here and now and that, in the words of the Greek philosopher Protagoras, man is the measure of all things. The important point is that morality is about how we behave whatever our world view. When The Guardian referred[1] in 2014 to Lord Falconer's bill creating a new moral landscape, it was not making a specifically religious point.

[1] See Page 24

We need to be clear too what is meant by the term 'religion'. The word tends to be used loosely to describe a system of belief and worship, but in its origins it means simply a restraining force - something that binds or inhibits us from doing what, left to ourselves, we might well do. The connection with belief and worship is obvious: if you hold certain things to be true as regards this life and what may lie beyond it, it is to be expected that that will govern your conduct - though, sadly, we can all think of examples where that is not evident in practice. But a religion is a consequence of a belief, not the belief itself. On this basis it might be argued that, for example, humanism is a religion but one that rests on a secular appreciation of the world rather than on a transcendental one.

In what follows we use the words 'religion' and 'religious' with their popular meanings, but it is important to be clear that there is a distinction to be drawn between our perceptions of reality (which, for those with a transcendental outlook, we may loosely call a 'faith') and religion (meaning our code of ethics, which may or may not derive from a faith).

Religion and Assisted Dying

Most of the faiths have adopted an opposing stance to legalisation. In September 2015 a statement from more than twenty faith leaders was published in The Guardian[2] expressing concerns about Rob Marris MP's 'assisted dying' bill. The signatories included the Archbishop of Canterbury, the Cardinal Archbishop of Westminster, the Free Churches Moderator, the Chief Rabbi, the Secretary-General of the Muslim Council of Britain, the Secretary of the Methodist Conference and the Director of the Network of Sikh Organisations in the UK.

---

[2] The Guardian, 5 September 2015

In fact, the joint statement made little reference to faith or religion. It focused predominantly on social values and it drew attention to the practical risks of a change in the law. "*Our concern*", it stated, "*is rooted in a profoundly human and profoundly sacred calling to care for the most vulnerable in our society, a concern shared by people of all faiths and none*"

The faith leaders noted that "*in the UK some 500,000 elderly people are abused each year, most by family members, often for financial reasons*" and that "*a change in the law would result, not in greater comfort, but in an added burden to consider ending their lives prematurely, a burden they ought not to be asked to bear*".

Supporters of 'assisted dying' say that faith groups are out of step with a majority of their adherents. For example, a group called Inter-Faith Leaders for Dignity in Dying (IFDiD), which is affiliated to the campaigning group Dignity in Dying (DiD), states on its website that *"there are many who are both committed worshippers and believe strongly that assisted dying should be available as a choice for terminally ill people"*. According to IFDiD:

> *"A YouGov survey commissioned by IFDiD found that 62% of people who identified as belonging to a religion supported the legalisation of assisted dying for terminally ill adults with mental capacity, whether they would want the choice for themselves or not. Only 18% were opposed"*[3].

Closer inspection of the poll raises doubts over this confident assertion. First, let us look at the question posed. It was this:

> "*Currently it is illegal for a doctor to help someone with a terminal illness to control their death, even if the person is suffering unbearably and is of sound mind. A new assisted dying law would mean that a terminally ill adult would have the option to control the time of their death with help from a doctor who would write a prescription for life-ending medication providing that they met*

---

[3] https://www.dignityindying.org.uk/take-action/religious-support/

> *upfront safeguards to determine whether they were likely to die within six months, are of sound mind and were informed of all their care and treatment options.*
>
> *"Whether or not you would want the choice for yourself, to what extent do you support or oppose the legislation of assisted dying for individuals of sound mind with terminal illnesses, subject to upfront safeguards?"*[4]

As with the more general opinion poll discussed in Chapter Three, the wording of this question is potentially misleading. It is not "*illegal for a doctor to help someone with a terminal illness to control his or her death*". A doctor is able to help the patient to control the process of dying by the prescription or administration of analgesics or other symptom-relieving medicines. If the patient wishes to allow nature to take its course and to die, the doctor has a professional duty to support that process with end-of-life care. The only thing a doctor may not legally - and ethically - do is to act in such a way as deliberately to bring about the patient's death. The first sentence of the question, however, conveys the false impression that the law is interfering unreasonably in medical care of the dying. That is untrue.

The new parliamentary bill to which the question refers would, we are told, allow *'help from a doctor*'. What could be more reassuring! So what help is implied? The doctor would *'write a prescription*'. Fair enough: that is something that doctors do. A prescription for what? The term used is 'life-ending medication'. This is a misuse of language. The term 'medication' implies treatment. The lethal drugs which would be prescribed under an 'assisted dying' regime have no therapeutic properties whatever. Their sole purpose is to bring about death. But the term 'medication' has a caring and benevolent flavour.

---

[4] You Gov Dignity in Dying Survey, Fieldwork 22-24 April 2013

We are told there would be 'upfront safeguards'. What safeguards? The bill to which the question refers contained no concrete safeguards. It included simply a handful of broadly-worded conditions for assisted suicide - a settled intent to die, mental capacity, freedom from coercion or duress - but it placed no requirement on a doctor considering a request to take any minimum steps to ensure that those conditions were met.

Now let us turn to the responses to this question. If we look at detailed analysis of the results rather than just at the headline figures, we see that the 62 per cent who are said to support legalisation actually consists of 27 per cent who 'strongly support' and 35 per cent who 'tend to support'. These results are not at all surprising. We are dealing with a complex and emotive subject of which large numbers of people have little knowledge or experience; and they are being asked to express an opinion by responding to a question the wording of which is potentially misleading. The question put to them is expressed in terms which are likely to appeal to any decent-minded citizen and to resonate with anyone who does not understand what is the legal position with regard to medical care of the dying or who has not read the parliamentary bill in question.

Further detailed analysis of the results also calls into question the description of the respondents as 'belonging to a religion'. Religious belief covers a range of positions, from (at one end of the spectrum) the devout and committed believer to (at the other end) someone who has no clearly defined faith but a general feeling that religion in its broadest sense is something to which he or she might subscribe. If we look at the breakdown of the responses in the survey we see that strong support for a change in the law was weakest among those who said they attended places of worship regularly and stronger among those who said they less frequently attended services. Of course, attendance at places of worship is not the only criterion of religious belief. But in terms of measurable data the conclusion that a substantial majority of the faith community supports a change in the law is open to question.

Campaigners for ‘assisted dying’ point to eminent churchmen, such as former Archbishop of Canterbury Lord Carey and Archbishop Desmond Tutu, who say they support a change in the law. It is normal in any organisation or group to find individuals who dissent from agreed teachings or policies. Their views are to be respected and listened to. They are, however, in a small minority. That does not make them wrong: there is an important role for dissent in any community. But nor does their eminence make them right.

It is undoubtedly the case that support for legalisation of 'assisted dying' extends into the faith community. However, this would come as a surprise only to those who see the issue of legalisation as predominantly a faith issue. In reality that is not the case. People with a religious faith are often people who have a strong disposition to compassion and are perhaps more susceptible to the compassionate terms in which the case for legalisation is presented. It is all too easy in such circumstances to lose sight of the essential issue in the 'assisted dying' debate, which is not whether or not such acts are compassionate but whether they should be licensed by law.

But, it may be argued, does not the existence of support for legalisation among some of the faith community indicate that the churches and other faith groups are out of step in this matter with their congregations? That may perhaps be so, but it raises the question of why the faith groups exist. They would probably say that they exist to teach and guide their flocks. If the latter do not accept what is being taught, that is a matter for them. But to suggest that the churches and other faith groups should adapt what they teach to what their adherents are apparently prepared to accept surely calls into question their *raison d’etre*.

It is also suggested that in speaking out in opposition to legalisation of 'assisted dying' the faith groups are seeking to impose their views on society as a whole. If this were true, it would be a serious charge. No group in society should be able to impose its views on the rest of us. But it is not true. What the churches and other faith groups are doing is giving to their flocks specifically, and to the public generally, their perspective of the issue. We may not concur with that perspective and, if that is so, we are at liberty to ignore it. But the suggestion that in giving their perspective the churches and other faith groups are imposing it on the rest of us is nonsense. Indeed, the allegation bears a striking resemblance to the cry, also heard from campaigners for legalisation, that the Medical Colleges and the BMA should not express a collective view but should stand back from and be neutral in the 'assisted dying' debate. In both cases they are giving us the benefit of their knowledge and experience. Parliament and the public are free to disregard what they say but it is unacceptable to seek to muzzle them because what they say is inconvenient.

But do the churches not have a privileged position in the shape of the 26 Anglican bishops who sit in the House of Lords? There are over 800 Peers in the Upper Chamber of Parliament. If this were a marginal issue and if all the bishops voted against legalisation, it is (just) conceivable that that might tip the scales. In reality that is far from being the case. If we look at the two occasions in recent years when proposals to legalise assisted suicide in one form or another have been put to a vote[5] in the House of Lords, we see that legalisation was rejected by substantial majorities, that only some of the bishops voted and that their votes represented a very small part of those majorities. The bishops, it would seem, take considerable care not to wield their influence *en bloc*.

---

[5] 12 May 2006 (Lord Joffe's 2005 Assisted Dying for the Terminally Ill Bill) and 7 July 2009 (Lord Falconer's Amendment to the Coroner's and Justice Bill)

There is, in any case, a wider issue to be noted here. If Peers, MPs or members of the public oppose legalisation and have religious beliefs, it does not follow that their opposition rests on those beliefs. It is not the case that people with a religious faith think and act entirely in religious terms. It is perfectly possible to have a faith-based objection to something but to have other objections to it as well which would exist without the faith factor. The 'assisted dying' debate is a good example of this phenomenon. Certainly for some people it has a faith dimension, but it has a number of other sides to it also - medical ethics, public safety and social messaging, for example - which raise serious doubts in the minds of many people, whether they have a religious faith or not. It is simplistic to see society as divided into two distinct camps - the supposed faith and secular communities. In reality, most people are a complex mixture of the two.

Secular Concepts

A number of secular concepts feature in the 'assisted dying' debate. Let us look at four of the most common - dignity, compassion, autonomy and the sanctity of life.

Dignity

Campaigners for legalisation want some people to be able to seek assistance with suicide in order to die with dignity. That is a laudable purpose. But it raises the question: what is meant by dying with dignity? Oregon's law explicitly equates physician-assisted suicide with dying with dignity, not only in its title but in its provisions. It states, for example, that "*in order to receive a prescription for medication to end his or her life in a humane and dignified manner, a qualified patient shall have made an oral request and a written request*"[6]. A doctor can write a prescription

---

[6] DWDA, Section 127.840, sub-section 3.06

for lethal drugs. Whether a doctor can guarantee that the result will be a humane and dignified death is something else.

Our dignity is our worth, but that immediately raises the question: in whose eyes? It is possible to look at this from a subjective or an objective standpoint. The subjective view is that we alone, as individuals, can judge whether or not we have dignity. In other words, our dignity is our sense of <u>self</u>-worth. So, for example, if we are seriously ill or incapacitated and have to be hoisted in and out of bed or taken to the lavatory, some might see such dependence on others as an infringement of their dignity because it causes them embarrassment and detracts from their ability to live independent lives. Indeed, the word 'independence' is encountered frequently in the 'assisted dying' debate. Giving evidence in 2004 to the Mackay Committee, an Oregon psychiatrist who had studied the motivations of people seeking legalised assisted suicide referred to "*seemingly unbearable situations where they have to rely on other people*" and to statements that "*they find being cared for intolerable*"[7].

This subjective view of dignity is easy to understand and to relate to. Others might argue, however, that there is a difference between our sense of dignity and dignity itself, and that our worth is determined by what we are rather than what we perceive ourselves to be. This perspective of dignity is perhaps more likely to be held by people with a transcendental world view. They might argue that, whatever our sense of self-worth at any particular moment, our true worth is our worth in the eyes of God. It is not, however, an exclusively faith-based perspective. Many people without a religious faith take the view that as human beings we have a status or worth that is in some way special.

Such perceptions may understandably cut little ice with seriously ill people who feel they have lost their dignity. They may see them as

[7] House of Lords Report 86-II (Session 2004-05), Page 289

platitudinous, if not patronising. However, there is an important practical issue here. In deciding whether or not we have dignity we do not start with a clean sheet of paper. Judgements of our self-worth can reflect how we are regarded or treated by others. If we are treated unkindly or dismissively, it is easy to feel that we are of little worth. Not everyone fits the stereotype of the no-nonsense man or woman who believes that his or her dignity is infringed by being dependent on others. Many seriously ill people are not so strong-willed or self-reliant: they can easily come to see themselves as of little worth as a result of they way they see others perceiving or treating them.

It is important to remember that dignity is more than a personal concept. It is not just a one-dimensional quality that we assert but something that we share with those around us. It is a concept that applies to us as a community, as much to people giving care and support as to those receiving it. That is, after all, what the word 'community' literally means - an exchange or sharing of services.

Compassion

Compassion is a key watchword of the campaign for legalisation. 'Assisted dying' is presented as a means of ending the suffering of terminally ill people. One of the campaigning slogans in the run-up to the most recent parliamentary debate on legalisation of 'assisted dying' was that "*no more would die but fewer would suffer*". Who would argue with the relief of suffering?

We need to begin by asking what we mean by suffering. It is easy to run away with the idea that what we are talking about here is pain and other physiological distress. The reality is more complex than that. One doctor who specialised in care of the dying put it this way to the Mackay Committee:

> "*I would certainly not suggest that palliative care can in all circumstances relieve all suffering...Within existing law doctors do*

seem confident, however, that physical symptoms can be treated in the last few weeks of life"

He believed that "*existential suffering and the fear of dependence may be much more relevant to requests for assisted dying than uncontrolled symptoms*"[8].

The same point was made by other experts, and in its report the committee referred to terminally ill people "*whose suffering derives more from the fact of their terminal illness and from the loss of control which this involves than from the symptoms of their disease*"[9].

The official annual reports coming out of Oregon reinforce the point. As we have observed in an earlier chapter, one of the main reasons which people who resort to that State's physician-assisted suicide law give for doing so is a "*decreasing ability to participate in activities that made life enjoyable*". It is completely understandable that a terminal illness and its accompanying restrictions on lifestyle should cause frustration and suffering of this kind. But the existential nature of much of the suffering associated with 'assisted dying' is often not made clear when the case for legalisation is presented. This tends to focus on physiological suffering, to which most people can easily relate but which modern medicine can to a large extent relieve or mitigate.

It is also arguable that for some seriously-ill people legalisation of physician-assisted suicide has the potential to increase rather than diminish their suffering. Under the law that we have, the option of obtaining lethal drugs to end one's life is not available. Some may see that as a denial of choice. But it is necessary to look at the other side of the coin. One person's choice can be another's burden. A specialist in end-of-life care giving evidence to the Mackay Committee referred to "*being faced with a constant choice*

---

[8] House of Lords Report 86-II (Session 2004-05), Page 552

[9] House of Lords Report 86-I (Session 2004-05), Paragraph 244

for the last months of your life as to whether you ought to opt for assisted suicide". It would, she suggested, "*be an increase in suffering because of the agonising choice which they are constantly presented with*"[10].

Often in life the hardest things to deal with are not what Shakespeare called the slings and arrows of outrageous fortune but rather the near-impossible decisions and dilemmas with which we are sometimes confronted. It is easy to dismiss this as paternalism, but it is important to remember that we are talking about presenting life-or-death choices to people who are in many cases under considerable mental and emotional stress. The highly determined man or woman who has been accustomed to a life of control may not find that too burdensome, but that is not the situation of most people who are faced with a terminal prognosis and are struggling to come to terms with the prospect of dying.

Autonomy

Another key word in the 'assisted dying' lexicon is autonomy. The argument is that how and when we die is a matter for us and for us alone: it is a choice that we should be able to make for ourselves provided that in doing so we do not cause harm to anyone else. It was expressed like this by the British Humanist Association in written evidence to the Mackay Committee:

> "*Humanists defend as important ethical principles the right of each individual to live by her/his own personal values and the freedom to make decisions about her/his own life so long as this does not result in harm to others. Humanists do not share some of the attitudes to death and dying held by some religious believers, in particular that the manner and time of death are for a deity to decide and/or that interference in the course of nature is unacceptable. The vast majority of humanists believe that we should have the choice of deciding these matters for ourselves, as*

---

[10] House of Lords Report 86-II (Session 2004-05), Page 555

do the general public. A clear request to die with dignity is a rational choice when the postponement of an inevitable and imminent death can offer no benefit to the sufferer. This is a situation where personal autonomy is clearly important and does no harm to others"[11].

There are some questionable assumptions made here - for example, that the law does not allow us to decide when to die or that dying with dignity can be equated with dying by assisted suicide. But, taken as a whole, the statement is an easy one to understand and it would probably resonate with many people.

However, the notion of personal autonomy that underlies it is open to question. Professor Onora O'Neill has expressed the point well:

"The original use of the term 'autonomy' was jurisprudential. The ancient Greeks contrasted colonies, whose laws were made for them by their mother cities, with self-legislating or autonomous cities that were not colonies but rather made their own laws. Autonomous cities were politically independent. This political or constitutional use of the term 'autonomy' is still current. It is quite different from contemporary understandings of individual autonomy, and the Greeks would not have spoken of individuals (who do not make laws at all) either as autonomous or as lacking autonomy"[12].

It may perhaps be argued that, if the ancient Greeks defined autonomy in that way, that is no reason why the concept should not be expanded to include personal as well as political autonomy. But that raises the important question of where the individual sits in relation to the wider community, a question that lies at the heart of this whole debate. It may sound responsibly libertarian to suggest that we should be able to behave as we wish provided that in doing so we do not cause harm to others. But who is to make

[11] House of Lords Report 86-II (Session 2004-05), Page 510

[12] Address to the Royal Society of Medicine 2010

these judgements as to the harmlessness of individual actions? Such decisions cannot surely be left to the person who is taking the action and has a vested interest in overlooking the collateral harm which may result from it. We all make judgements every day about whether our actions will impact on other people, and experience shows that many of those judgements are made, whether thoughtlessly or maliciously, without serious regard for the interests of others.

The argument that we should be free to behave as we wish provided that we do not harm others in the process does not of itself provide a serious basis for changing the law. If the law were to be changed, our legislators would have to address the question of whether, and if so how, it might be possible to balance the rights of the individual against those of the wider community. This raises the all-important issue of public safety, which is addressed in Chapter Seven.

It is in any case arguable that what is at issue here is not a simple extension of autonomy. An 'assisted dying' law would not enable people to end their own lives but to seek assistance from doctors to enable them to do that. As we have noted in an earlier chapter, the right that is being sought is not a right to die, which exists already, but a right to involve someone else in bringing about our deaths.

Sanctity of Life

The term 'sanctity of life' is often assumed to have religious connotations. In fact, sanctity simply means inviolability. It is nonetheless true that sanctity of life tends to be raised as an argument against changing the law, and some of those who raise it do indeed raise it in a faith context.

It is arguable that society does not believe in the absolute inviolability of human life. We used to have the death penalty, our armed forces may legally kill in war and the police may use lethal force in self-defence or to protect another whose life is believed to be at risk.

These are, however, fundamentally different concepts from that of 'assisted dying'. The death penalty was intended as a measure of social protection. It did, however, generate a good deal of opposition, though not so much, perhaps, because it involved the termination of a life but because it did so in what to many seemed an unnatural and sadistic manner - giving notice to the convicted person that he or she would be hanged at a particular time on a specific date. It was also not free from error. Despite exhaustive judicial process there were cases when, it has been suggested, the wrong person was hanged. It is the (much increased) risk of error that worries many of the opponents of 'assisted dying'.

Killing in war and self-defence (or to protect others) is also different in concept from 'assisted dying'. We do not send soldiers to war in order to kill but to defend their country: a soldier who kills on the battlefield is not guilty of murder. A police officer who shoots an armed law-breaker is not trying to bring about the death of the other person but to maintain the law or to protect himself or another person whose life is threatened. It is possible to argue about whether specific wars are justified on grounds of national defence or whether minimum force has been used in a particular confrontation on the streets. But the principle is clear, and it is one that most people can understand.

By contrast, handing lethal drugs to someone to enable him or her to commit suicide has only one aim in view - to bring about the death of a specific person. It is possible to argue that here too the death of the person is simply the means and that there is a higher end, such as the relief of suffering. But the validity of such an argument depends on whether there are other, less drastic, ways of relieving the suffering (the equivalent of the minimum-force test) and just what the suffering consists of. In individual cases these tests might conceivably be passed. But, as has been argued in an earlier chapter, there is a difference between accepting that an act may be illegal but morally justifiable in individual cases and licensing such acts by law in advance and in prescribed circumstances.

One of the parallels that is often drawn with 'assisted dying' is that of compassionate euthanasia for animals. It is common to hear the refrain that 'you wouldn't let a dog suffer like this', the inference being that we should be able to put humans out of their misery on request. We need to remember, however, that while most people who take their pets to be put down do so for compassionate reasons there are some who do so from other motives - for example, because the animals concerned are a nuisance or they are tired of looking after them or they have become too expensive to maintain. If there is a parallel between 'assisted dying' and veterinary euthanasia, it is not the one that is sometimes supposed.

In Conclusion

It is possible to mount respectable moral cases both for changing and for maintaining the existing law. Concepts such as dignity, compassion and autonomy are common currency to both sides of the debate.

There are some themes which run through this narrative. One is the need to respect the moral standpoints of those who disagree with us. In a predominantly secular society it is all too easy to marginalise the faith perspective of 'assisted dying' and to suggest that in opposing a change in the law the faith groups are seeking to impose religious views on the rest of society. A moment's reflection shows that this accusation is groundless. We should all be free to express our insights into this complex and controversial issue, whatever those insights might be. Indeed, it is arguable that we have a civic duty to do so. It is facile to suggest that those who have a moral objection to 'assisted dying' need not avail themselves of it and should therefore stand back from the debate as to whether it should be legalised for others. To stand aside and say nothing when we fear that mistaken decisions may be taken is tantamount to passing by on the other side. In a free society we have a duty as well as a right to speak out.

Equally, the opponents of legalisation need to recognise that they do not have a monopoly of the moral case. The case for changing the law is rooted in honourable and laudable instincts, such as a wish to spare terminally ill people suffering as they die, and it can be defended by reference to decent humanitarian principles. It is necessary also to recognise that society has changed considerably over the last few decades and that there is a need to engage with this debate, as with others, in terms which the public understand. Too often that does not happen.

Most people, whether they support or oppose legalisation, appear to be agreed on one thing - that, if there ever were to be legislation authorising doctors to supply lethal drugs to seriously ill people, it would need to be surrounded with the strictest of safeguards. In other words, this debate is not only about personal morality but also - and, many would argue, primarily - about public safety. In the next chapter we ask the question: just how safe is safe?

Chapter Seven

A Matter of Public Safety

Ilora Finlay and Robert Preston

Salus Populi Suprema Lex[1]

We come now to examining the practicalities of implementing an 'assisted dying' law. We examine what safeguards have been proposed for such legislation in Britain, how realistic they are and how much protection they might give to vulnerable people. The basic question we are asking here is: just how safe is safe?

The Principle of Safety

In any sphere of activity we can have as much or as little safety as we like or as we think appropriate. However, there is a principle which commands broad agreement - that the degree of safety accorded to something should be commensurate with the degree of risk or the consequences of failure. Thus, we have more rigorous safety systems in cars than on bicycles and in aircraft than in cars. In the same way railway signals are designed to default to red in the event of a malfunction.

An assisted suicide law is, by any definition, high on - if not at the top of - any risk register. The consequences of error are, quite literally, deadly and they are also irreparable. It follows that the safeguards to be built into any legislation permitting such a

[1] 'Public safety is the most important law', a thesis widely accepted as one of the fundamental principles of law-making

practice must be very stringent indeed. The fact that we are talking about actions to be performed at the request and with the consent of the victim (to borrow the word used in the Crown Prosecution Service's policy for prosecutors) does not alter this. Safety measures are frequently put in place to prevent people not only from harming others but also from harming themselves as a result of willing actions.

It is also important to remember that we are talking about decisions which would have to be taken at a highly stressful time - when the people taking them are terminally ill and struggling to come to terms with their illness and with the prospect of death - and that such things as depression or a feeling of obligation to others have the potential to distort judgement.

What are the safeguards?

Safeguards for 'assisted dying' legislation need to meet three broad requirements. They must designate accurately and without ambiguity those groups of people who are to be made eligible to receive assistance to end their lives; they must place decision-making in such cases in the hands of persons who are qualified to make the difficult judgements that are involved; and they must put in place robust procedures both to assist and to audit the decision-making process.

So, what are the safeguards proposed? There seems to be general agreement among those who are pressing for legislation of this nature in Britain that 'assisted dying' should be made available to people who are terminally ill, mentally competent and acting voluntarily and without pressure and that the request should reflect a settled wish to die. There is also an assumption that it should be doctors who should consider such requests, decide whether or not whether they meet the criteria and, if so, supply the required drugs. Some of the more recent proposals have included a requirement for a judge of the Family Division of the High Court to confirm a doctor's decision.

The Decision-Making Process

It is fair to ask why doctors should be considered to have any role to play in actions which are not normally seen as part of health care. Doctors certainly have a part to play if the desire is to link 'assisted dying' to specific clinical states. In that case someone with the appropriate knowledge and experience has to confirm that an applicant for assistance to end his or her life has the designated clinical condition and that the prognosis falls within any time limits which are set. But that is not the same thing as assessing whether the conditions for 'assisted dying' as a whole are met. As we have observed above, most of these conditions, including whether a request for 'assisted dying' stems from a settled wish to die and whether a request is truly voluntary, raise personal or social rather than medical questions and it is doubtful whether many doctors are in a position to form a judgement about them which goes beyond what the patient has told them.

In Chapter Two we referred to a 2015 survey of 1,000 GPs in Britain which revealed that only 14 per cent would be prepared to conduct a full assessment of a request for legalised 'assisted dying'. In the same survey 39 per cent of respondents answered in the affirmative when asked whether they would be willing to "*conduct a basic assessment of the requesting patient's eligibility (for example, give your opinion to the patient's primary assessor on prognosis and involvement of palliative services)*". In other words, while only one in seven respondents was willing to conduct a full assessment, nearly four out of ten said they might be willing to provide strictly-medical advice to someone charged with making a decision about overall eligibility. While this hardly suggests substantial support among doctors for legalisation, it does indicate a perception that there is a difference between doctors giving advice on matters which are within their professional competence and requiring them to act as the gatekeepers of an 'assisted dying' regime.

So, if the decisions are not to be made by doctors, who is to make them? In 2014 the Supreme Court rejected an Appeal which sought to allow doctors to administer voluntary euthanasia in a specific case. In giving the Judgment the President of the Court speculated on how, if the law were to be changed, giving rights to some might be balanced against protecting others from harm. He expressed the view that "*there is much to be said for the idea...that it should be a High Court judge who decides the issue*" and that "*it may well be that the risks to the weak and vulnerable could be eliminated or reduced to an acceptable level if no assistance could be given to a person who wishes to die unless and until a Judge of the High Court has been satisfied that his wish to do so was voluntary, clear, settled and informed*".

He continued:

> "*Over the past twenty-five years the High Court has been able to sanction a number of actions in relation to people which will lead to their deaths or will represent serious invasions of their body - sterilisation, denial of treatment, withdrawal of artificial nutrition and hydration, switching off a life-support machine, and surgery causing death to preserve the life of another*"[2].

The suggestion was taken up by Lord Falconer in his Assisted Dying Bill of June 2015 and has been repeated in his Private Member Bill tabled in January 2020[3]. These bills proposed that assistance with suicide might be given to a person who had been considered to meet certain criteria (eg terminal illness, capacity to make the decision, a settled and voluntary wish) '*subject to the consent of*

---

[2] R (on the application of Nicklinson and another)(Appellants) v Ministry of Justice (Respondents); R (on the application of AM)(AP)(Respondent) v The Director of Public Prosecutions (Appellant) [2014] UKSC38, Paragraphs 123-124

[3] HL Bill 69 (Session 2020-21)

the High Court (Family Division)"[4]. An almost identical Assisted Dying No.2 Bill presented to the House of Commons by Rob Marris MP in 2015 made the same provision[5]. As observed above, Mr Marris's bill was rejected by the House of Commons.

In what follows we take Lord Falconer's latest (2020) bill as illustrating what the 'assisted dying' lobby believes to be appropriate in regard to decision-making. Notwithstanding its reference to the High Court, the bill continues to place responsibility on doctors for overall decision-making. It provides that, before an application may be made to the High Court, two doctors must be "*satisfied*" not only that the applicant is terminally ill but also "*has the capacity to make the decision to end their own life; and has a clear and settled intention to end their own life which has been reached voluntarily, on an informed basis and without coercion or duress*[6]. In other words, responsibility for overall decision-making remains with doctors and the role of the Court is to confirm the decision.

While some might perhaps see the involvement of the Court as an additional safeguard, in reality it suffers from the weakness of dividing responsibility for the same decision. The Association for Palliative Medicine (APM) explained the point with clarity in 2015 when the same proposal appeared in Lord Falconer's bill of that year. It stated:

> "*We welcome the requirement to involve the High Court, but we believe it is insufficient and potentially confusing to divide responsibility for the same decision between doctors and the Court. It has the potential to produce situations in which each party to an assisted suicide decision takes spurious comfort from the involvement of the other and no one is fully accountable for the outcome*".

The APM continued:

---

[4] HL Bill 25 (Session 2015-16), Clause 1(1)

[5] Bill 7 (Session 2015-16), Clause 1(3)

[6] Bill 69 (Session 2020-21), Clause 3(3)

> "*Doctors' expertise lies in diagnosis of illness, in estimating its likely course and in managing its effects. Dispassionate consideration of complex issues - such as the settled nature of a request for assisted suicide, the weight of personal or domestic issues that may be influencing the request and the person's capacity to make such a serious and irreversible decision - is the proper province of the Court - and of the Court alone*"[7].

Involvement of the High Court is certainly a step forward in the 'assisted dying' debate. But, if the Court were to be the decision-maker rather than just a back-stop, it would need to handle requests for 'assisted dying' in the same way that it handles other life-or-death decisions. That would require the Court itself to investigate requests for 'assisted dying', seeking advice from those who are able and willing to contribute their expertise on specific aspects, including doctors, psychiatrists, social workers and persons who are familiar with or would be affected by the request, such as the applicant and his or her family members. The Court would then be responsible for making a decision based on the overall merits of the application. To put it another way, the role of doctors would be that of expert witnesses to the Court, a role they already perform in other contexts, not that of first-level judges.

Some suggest that requiring the High Court to investigate requests for assisted suicide is inappropriate. They argue that people wishing to have assistance to end their lives could find the legal processes intimidating, expensive and drawn-out. There may be some substance in this argument. But we should perhaps ask ourselves whether it is appropriate to seek to make such decisions easy. We would not wish to be misunderstood. We have no wish to impose unnecessary burdens on someone who is terminally ill. Our point is that such life-or-death decisions are grave and irrevocable. It is unlikely that anyone who is resolved and determined about seeking assistance to end his or her life and has

---

[7] Letter from the Association for Palliative Medicine to Members of the House of Lords 9 January 2015

a firmly settled wish to do so would be diverted from doing so by having to go the High Court. But there is perhaps something to be said for a process which might cause less serious applicants to pause and reflect.

Placing decision-making, whether solely or predominantly, with doctors does the opposite. It places 'assisted dying' within the comfort zone of health care. Whatever criticisms are levelled at the NHS in the media, there is no doubt that most people in Britain regard it in a benevolent light and they see doctors as people who will always act in their best interests. A decision by a doctor that a request for 'assisted dying' should proceed, even if subject to Court endorsement, conveys the potentially misleading message that ending the patient's life is a best-interests procedure.

This is not to say that investigation and decision-making by the Court is infallible. We all of us bring our own experiences and prejudices to assessing situations. But the Court may be said to have some advantages over other potential assessors. One of these is that, as the President of the Supreme Court observed, it is accustomed to investigating and taking decisions on other life-or-death issues. Another is that its members, though human like the rest of us, are trained and experienced in objective and dispassionate analysis of the facts, in seeking and weighing expert opinion from a wide range of fields and in balancing the rights of individuals against those of society. If we were ever to have an 'assisted dying' law in Britain, there can be little doubt that the High Court route is probably the safest one to follow so far as decision-making is concerned. But it would need to be a Court-led rather than a Court-endorsed process and it would need to limit the involvement of doctors to the role of expert witnesses on matters within their professional competence rather than turn them into first-level arbiters.

Diagnosis and Prognosis

The first requirement in designing any safeguards for legalised 'assisted dying' is to define accurately and without ambiguity those groups of people to whom it is to be offered. The 'assisted dying' bills we have seen in Britain generally focus on terminal illness as a key qualifying condition. But just what is 'terminal illness'? According to Lord Falconer's 2020 Private Member Bill, a terminal illness is "*an inevitably progressive condition which cannot be reversed by treatment*", as a consequence of which the patient "*is reasonably expected to die within six months*"[8]. This definition, which is a repetition of that contained in his 2015 bill, is similar to that which appears in Oregon's PAS law, which (as observed in Chapter Five) defines a terminal illness as "*an incurable and irreversible disease that has been medically confirmed and will, within reasonable medical judgement, produce death within six months*"[9].

While diagnosis of terminal illness is generally reliable, errors do occur. A patient who was referred to one of the authors nearly 30 years ago had been told by two doctors that he was terminally ill and had an estimated three months to live. He is alive today, nearly thirty years later. The Mackay Committee was told by the Royal College of Pathologists that post-mortems showed that *"significant errors (ie misdiagnosis of terminal illness resulting in inappropriate treatment) occur in around five per cent of cases"*[10]. More recently, Dr John Lee, a retired professor of pathology and former NHS consultant pathologist, has written that *"autopsy studies typically show major discrepancies between actual findings and clinical diagnosis in a quarter to a third of cases"*[11]. This is not

---

[8] Hl Bill 69 (Session 2020-21), Clause 2(1)

[9] DWDA, Section 127.800, Subsection 1.01 (12)

[10] House of Lords Report 86-II (Session 2004-05), Page 730

[11] The Spectator, 30 May 2020, Page 16

to suggest that diagnosis as a process is unreliable but that errors do occur and rather more often than might be imagined.

If diagnosis can occasionally get it wrong, prognosis is more vulnerable to error. Though we are accustomed to hearing phrases such as 'three months to live', in reality forecasting life expectancy in terminal illness is far from being an exact science. The Mackay Committee was told by a doctor from the Royal College of General Practitioners that, while it is possible to make reasonably accurate prognoses of death within minutes, hours or a few days, *"when this stretches to months, then the scope for error can extend into years"*[12]. A doctor from the Royal College of Physicians agreed. *"Prognosticating may be better when somebody is within the last two or three weeks of their life"*, he said. But, he added, *"I have say that, when they are six or eight months away from it, it is actually pretty desperately hopeless as an accurate factor"*.[13]

In fact, it is not only at ranges such as six months that problems of prognosis arise. Baroness Neuberger's review of the Liverpool Care Pathway, which addressed the prognosis and treatment of patients considered to be in the last hours and days of life, commented that "*there are no precise ways of telling accurately when a patient is in the last days of life*" and that "*more research is needed into improving the accuracy of these [prognostic] tools, where possible; and, where it is not, clear guidance and training is needed for doctors and MDT [multi-disciplinary teams] on understanding and explaining the uncertain timings within the dying process*"[14].

It is important to recognise these uncertainties because a patient diagnosed with a terminal illness will understandably be anxious to know 'how long have I got' and because a perception of life expectancy is likely to be an important factor in a decision to seek

[12] House of Lords Report 86-I (Session 2004-05), Paragraph 118

[13] Ibid

[14] 'More Care. Less Pathway', An Independent Review of the Liverpool Care Pathway, 2014

'assisted dying'. Yet prognosis over months rather than weeks is often not recognised as being in many cases little more than a best guess.

However, there is another problem with these definitions of terminal illness apart from that of unreliable prognosis. They derive from a mistaken belief that a terminal illness is necessarily an incurable condition which results in an early death. When we think of terminal illness, we tend to think of cancer or other conditions with a relatively-short trajectory between diagnosis and death - though with modern diagnostic and treatment regimes survival periods for cancer are increasing year by year. This is a misapprehension. There are many people with a range of incurable but chronic illnesses, such as MS or Parkinson's disease or heart disease, with which given careful management they can live for many years - in some cases for decades. These and other chronic illnesses are 'inevitably progressive conditions' - or, to quote from Oregon's law, 'incurable and irreversible diseases'. They can have an up-and-down trajectory, with successive periods of decline and recovery, and it would be perfectly possible for a doctor to say, at one of the illness's low points, that the patient could be "reasonably expected" to die within six months.

Consider also an elderly patient with a number of incurable co-morbidities, such as diabetes or heart disease or high blood pressure, none of which individually can be considered terminal but the combination of which, taken together with the patient's advanced years, could well justify a judgement that the patient concerned could be "reasonably expected" to die within six months.

In other words, what appears at first sight to be a bill restricted to a small group of people designated as terminally ill and close to dying can be seen, on closer inspection, to embrace larger numbers of chronically ill people as well as others who are of an age and general medical condition where death might be expected in the near future. The report on PAS deaths in Oregon in 2019 states that around 3.2 per cent of those who ended their lives by legalised assisted suicide in that year had been suffering from what it calls 'other illnesses'. This category, according to a footnote, *"includes deaths due to arthritis, arteritis, blood disease, complications from a fall, kidney failure, musculoskeletal system disorders, sclerosis and stenosis"*[15].

It is against this background that we have to look critically at statements to the effect that 'assisted dying' for the terminally ill would have a very restricted catchment area. Take, for example, Lord Falconer's statement in the House of Lords in 2014 that *"disabled or older people without a terminal illness would not be eligible for an assisted death"*[16]. In the real world there is not something called 'terminal illness' which is distinct from disability or old age. These states often overlap with each other. Large numbers of people, some of them with disabilities and many of them elderly, suffer from chronic and incurable illnesses of one sort or another. It is this failure to see the inter-connections that worries many elderly or disabled people about how an 'assisted dying' law could be interpreted in practice.

Settled Intent

Here we come to a question of great importance in assessing a request for assisted suicide. Is the request the result of mature consideration by the person concerned? Or is it a depressive and transient response to receiving a diagnosis of serious illness? Decisions of this nature, if followed through, are irrevocable and there is consensus on both sides of the debate that, where there is a possibility of second thoughts, a request should not be allowed to proceed. Hence the requirement that a request for assisted

[15] Oregon Health Authority, Oregon Death with Dignity Act, 2019 Data Summary

[16] House of Lords Hansard 18 July 2014, Column 775

suicide should proceed from a settled intent. There is no dispute, therefore, over the aim of this safeguard.

The problem arises in reaching the required judgement. We have touched on this question briefly in earlier chapters and highlighted the difficulty that, where a doctor has only recently been introduced to a patient for the purpose of seeking assisted suicide (a circumstance likely to be common given the unwillingness of the majority of doctors to participate in such practices), it is next to impossible to make a knowledge-based judgement of how much thought has gone into the request. The proposals we have seen in England and Wales have ignored this problem. They have contented themselves with stating that a person seeking assisted suicide must have "*a clear and settled intention to end their own life*". Just how that judgement is to be made has not been explained.

Patrick Harvie MSP's Assisted Suicide (Scotland) Bill, which was rejected by the Scottish Parliament in 2015, adopted a different, and in some respects a more imaginative, approach to this question. It mandated a three-stage process of assessment of requests for assisted suicide in place of the two stages envisaged by campaigners south of the border. The first stage, known as a 'Preliminary Declaration', was to be completed before a request for assisted suicide could be made. It required a declaration to be signed that, "*if I become/am eligible to seek assistance to commit suicide that is made lawful by the Assisted Suicide (Scotland) Act 2014, I am willing to consider whether to request it*"[17]. In other words, people who thought that they might at some point in the future wish to consider seeking assistance with suicide if they found themselves in the circumstances envisaged in Mr Harvie's bill would be able to make a declaration to that effect if they so wished.

[17] Assisted Suicide (Scotland) Bill (SP Bill 40), Session 4 (2013), Schedule 1

The consultation document[18] which preceded Mr Harvie's bill described a preliminary declaration as "*a clear delineator between those who might wish an assisted suicide and others who do not*". It stated that, if a declaration had been on a patient's file "*for a period of time*", a doctor would be able "*to take this into consideration when looking at all the circumstances of a request for an assisted suicide*". This is an interesting concept. It is arguable that, if someone has taken the trouble to make a formal declaration to the effect that in certain circumstances he or she might wish to consider requesting lawful assistance with suicide and if that declaration has been on the patient's file "*for a period of time*", that might be seen as one indicator of a settled intent.

However, the potential value of this provision in Mr Harvie's Bill was negated by the requirement[19] that no more than a week need elapse between the making of a preliminary declaration and the filing of a request for assisted suicide. Such a qualification contributes nothing to resolving the difficult problem of how to separate requests which derive from a settled intent from others which have been reached without mature reflection. A preliminary declaration made twelve months before a request for assisted suicide might be interpreted as evidence of settled intent. But one week? The concept was an imaginative one but it was nullified by the proposed timescale.

It is, however, an issue to which those who campaign for a change in the law on either side of the border might wish to give further thought. They tell us that many people want to have the option of 'assisted dying' if and when they become terminally or otherwise seriously ill. It is surely not unreasonable, then, to suggest that those who feel like this and wish to be taken seriously if they should make such a request should make their wishes clear well in

---

[18] Assisted Dying (Scotland) Bill, Consultation Document, Pages 11 and 14

[19] Assisted Suicide (Scotland) Bill (SP Bill 40), Session 4 (2013), Section 8(3)(c)

advance and as a means of declaring that this is an issue to which they have given some thought and on which they have reached preliminary conclusions. Such a declaration could be withdrawn at any time and would carry with it no obligation to proceed with a request for assisted suicide. But it would provide at least a pointer towards the presence of a settled intent.

Whether many people would make such declarations in practice is open to question. It is not uncommon to hear people talk about not wanting to 'linger on' with a serious illness. It is doubtful, however, whether many of these are serious statements of intent. People frequently say they would not want to have cardio-pulmonary resuscitation or other life-saving interventions. Yet, as noted in Chapter Two, very few of us make Advance Decisions to Refuse Treatment, perhaps because the making of such declarations calls for a focusing of the mind. An advance declaration of a wish to consider legalised 'assisted dying' in certain circumstances might possibly have the same effect.

Capacity

The 'assisted dying' bills that have been presented in recent years to the Westminster Parliament require that a person seeking assistance with suicide must have "*the capacity to make the decision to end their own life*". They also say that "*capacity shall be construed in accordance with the Mental Capacity Act 2005*"[20]. So we need to start by looking at the Mental Capacity Act (MCA).

The MCA starts from the principle that "*a person must be assumed to have capacity unless it is established that he lacks capacity*" and that "*a person is not to be treated as unable to make a decision merely because he makes an unwise decision*"[21]. On the face of it, therefore, if the capacity of someone requesting assistance with

---

[20] See HL Bill 69 ISession 2020-21), Clause 12

[21] MCA Clause 1

suicide is to be judged in accordance with the MCA, it should be assumed that the person making the request has capacity unless there is good reason to believe he or she does not - even if it is believed that the request is unwise.

However, the Mental Capacity Act also states that "*for the avoidance of doubt, it is hereby declared that nothing in this Act is to be taken to affect the law relating to murder or manslaughter or the operation of section 2 of the Suicide Act 1961 (c. 60) (assisting suicide)*"[22]. In other words, the Act does not apply to requests for assistance with suicide or to acts done with the deliberate intention of ending another person's life. It was not designed for such situations.

As we have observed in a previous chapter, capacity is decision-specific. A person may have capacity to make some decisions - for example, about what to wear or eat or which film to go and see - but not others, such as having or refusing surgery. The degree of capacity required depends on the complexity and gravity of the decision in question. There can be few decisions more grave than a decision to take one's own life or to ask someone else to provide us with the means to take it.

The MCA defines an absence of capacity as follows:

> *"A person lacks capacity in relation to a matter if at the material time he is unable to make a decision for himself in relation to the matter because of an impairment of, or a disturbance in the functioning of, the mind or brain"*[23].

More specifically:

> *"A person is unable to make a decision for himself if he is unable—*
> *(a) to understand the information relevant to the decision,*
> *(b) to retain that information,*

---

[22] MCA Clause 62

[23] MCA, Clause 2(1)

(c) to use or weigh that information as part of the process of making the decision, or
(d) to communicate his decision (whether by talking, using sign language or any other means)"[24].

Assessing capacity is not, however, just a matter of establishing whether or not someone is *compos mentis* and able to make him- or herself understood. It is possible to have all our mental faculties intact but to have our judgement impaired either by a medical condition or by circumstances. The Mackay Committee was told that some people "*have episodes of reactive depression as a result of the diagnosis of a life-limiting illness*"[25] and that, while estimates varied, this was thought to affect 25-40 per cent of cancer patients. The committee was told of "*moderate to severe depression and anxiety at various stages throughout the course of many diseases*" and that "*measurement of these difficulties is problematic, particularly at the end of life, because many of the symptoms of depression are confounded by symptoms of disease*"[26].

The committee was also alerted to the problem of cognitive impairment affecting patients with neurological conditions. The Association of British Neurologists stated that:

> "*There are patients who to the lay public appear relatively normal but could have severe cognitive impairments and therefore would be unable to give informed decisions in an area such as this*"[27].

Against this expert background what tests do the 'assisted dying' proposals that we have seen propose in order to ensure that assisted suicide is offered only to people who are mentally competent? None. They require no more than that a doctor should

---

[24] MCA, Clause 3(1)
[25] House of Lords Report 86-I (Session 2004-05), Paragraph 124
[26] Idib
[27] Idib, Paragraph 125

be "*satisfied*" that an applicant for assisted suicide has "*the capacity to make the decision to end their own life*".

Oregon's assisted suicide law requires that:

> "*If in the opinion of the attending physician or the consulting physician*[28] *a patient may be suffering from a psychiatric or psychological disorder or depression causing impaired judgement, either physician shall refer the patient for counseling. No medication to end a patient's life in a humane and dignified manner*[29] *shall be prescribed until the person performing the counseling determines that the patient is not suffering from a psychiatric or psychological disorder or depression causing impaired judgement*"[30].

In his 2005 Assisted Dying for the Terminally Ill Bill Lord Joffe included a similar provision. This provision was, however, dropped from subsequent bills and did not reappear until Lord Falconer's 2015 Assisted Dying Bill, which required a doctor who had doubts as to the presence of mental capacity to refer an applicant for assisted suicide to "*an appropriate specialist*" and to "*take account of any opinion provided*". The same provision appears in Lord Falconer's 2020 bill[31].

This is certainly a welcome step forward. It is noteworthy, however, that what is proposed is that a doctor who has doubts about the presence of mental capacity should be required not to secure the agreement of the 'appropriate specialist' (whatever that

---

[28] The terms 'attending' and 'consulting' physician are used in Oregon's law to designate the first and second doctors, respectively, who agree to consider a request for assisted suicide

[29] The phrase to 'end life in a human and dignified manner' is a euphemism which appears in many places in Oregon's law to denote the provision of lethal drugs in order to assist suicide. It has no qualitative meaning.

[30] DWDA, Section 127.825, sub-section 3.03

[31] HL Bill 69, Clause 3(5)

term might mean) before proceeding to supply lethal drugs, but simply to '*take account of*' his or her '*opinion*'. In other words, it would be open to a non-specialist doctor to override the assessment of a specialist in capacity assessment.

That aside, we have to ask ourselves the question: is it enough to require doctors who agree to consider requests for assisted suicide to seek specialist help only in cases of doubt? As we have seen in Chapter Five, Oregon's 'if in doubt' procedure has been shown to fail: research has shown that some people who have ended their lives through legalised physician-assisted suicide had been suffering from clinical depression which had not been diagnosed by the doctors assessing them or referred for specialist evaluation and treatment.

It is not easy to see why there is so much resistance on the part of the 'assisted dying' lobby to the idea that specialist psychiatric assessment should be mandatory where requests are made for assistance with suicide. After all, expression of a suicide wish is normally regarded as grounds for either psychiatric assessment and treatment or at least careful exploration of what lies behind it. If a doctor encounters a patient who says he wishes to take his own life, the doctor has a professional duty of care to safeguard that patient from harm. So why should a request for assistance with suicide be seen differently?

One objection that is frequently heard is that mandatory referral would increase the number of hurdles which applicants for assisted suicide would have to clear, that it could add to their suffering and that it would lengthen the assessment process for people who do not have long to live. On this last point Lord Joffe told the Mackay Committee, *a propos* his own 'assisted dying' bill, that "*we are concerned, if there were so many steps...the patients will all have died before we get through them*"[32].

---

[32] House of Lords Report 86-II (Session 2004-05), Page 49

This argument, however, rests on an assumption - one that underlies much of the campaigning for legalisation of 'assisted dying' - that requests for assistance with suicide come from people who are clear and resolved in their thoughts and that to insist on careful exploration of those requests is as unnecessary as it is unkind. It discounts the possibility that some of those requests could come from people who have capacity issues which might not be immediately apparent to a generalist doctor, and especially to one with no prior knowledge of them as patients. It also fails to see that the primary purpose of the criminal law is to protect people, and especially the vulnerable, from harm - including self-harm - rather than to facilitate actions on which they may wish to embark.

There is perhaps an analogy here with the conduct of criminal trials. Some people are irritated by the seemingly-endless lengths to which the courts go to ensure that defendants receive a fair hearing. They assume that, if there is sufficient evidence to bring someone to trial, he or she is more than likely to be guilty. Yet the presumption of innocence is a cardinal feature of our justice system. As the jurist William Blackstone put it in the 1760s, it is better that ten guilty people escape than that one innocent should suffer. In the same way it is arguable that it is better that ten determined people seeking assisted suicide should be put to some additional inconvenience than that one vulnerable person should be put at risk.

A system of mandatory referral for psychological assessment has one other advantage which is often not recognised. It protects doctors who agree to assess requests for assisted suicide and have doubts about capacity from accusations, from applicants or their families, of foot-dragging. Anyone who thinks such situations could not occur should reflect that doctor-patient relationships are not invariably all sweetness and light: patients do sometimes get upset when doctors insist on tests or otherwise decline to fall in with their demands. Mandatory referral protects all parties.

Pressure

There is agreement on both sides of the 'assisted dying' debate that there must be no pressure to request assistance with suicide and that a person making such a request must be acting voluntarily. But it is not enough just to say that: the means have to be found to ensure that such pressures are not being brought to bear, which in turn requires that we understand from where those pressures might arise.

There are two kinds of pressure that might be at work where a person makes a request for assistance to take his or her own life. There are external and internal pressures. External pressure is where there are factors outside the person concerned which incline him or her to make such a request. Elderly people, for example, might come under pressure from their children or other relatives to take themselves off because they are a nuisance or because caring for them is becoming difficult or expensive. It is easy to discount such malicious pressure on the basis that we ourselves would not dream of behaving in that way and we cannot imagine others of our acquaintance doing so. But it is salutary to recall that there are an estimated 500,000 cases of elder abuse in Britain every year, the majority of which occur within families.

External pressure need not be overt or even maliciously intended. Subtle hints can be dropped. And, even when there is no intent to make the person being cared for feel uncomfortable, there can be signs of care fatigue - short temper, weariness and care-worn demeanour - which can all too easily be read as a wish that the person would die.

This brings us to the issue of internal pressure - namely, pressure that comes from within a person to 'do the decent thing' and relieve others of a care or a financial burden. The risk of this sort of situation arising is considerably greater than was once the case. As noted in Chapter Three, families are often not the cohesive units that they once were, and in today's world it is often the case that both partners must go out to work in order to keep their family's heads above water. In such circumstances a seriously-ill elderly relative who needs care can present major problems and it is not difficult to envisage a situation where an elderly parent might opt to hasten his or her death in order to remove a burden from a struggling family or to ensure that assets acquired during a lifetime are not consumed by being spent on paid care but can be handed on to the family intact.

There are some who have argued that there is nothing wrong with such self-sacrifice. Baroness Warnock put it this way when she spoke in support of Lord Falconer's Assisted Dying Bill in the House of Lords in July 2014:

> *"It is somchow thought to be wrong that people who are approaching death and are terminally ill should take into account the suffering, expense and misery they are causing to their family as they are being a burden. Of course, they are also a burden to the state. Why is it that this is thought to be a wrong motive, or part of a motive, for wanting to end one's life when it is coming to an end anyway...For all of one's life up to that stage, altruism is regarded as rather a good thing, a virtue. If one sacrifices oneself in a modest way for one's family, that is also thought virtuous. I do not understand why one should not be allowed to exercise that virtue at the very end of one's life, and not have it assumed that this is an idea that has been put into one's head by somebody else. It is not; it is there already"*[33].

The answer to Baroness Warnock's question is simple. It may well be a virtue in any individual case for someone to seek assisted suicide from the altruistic motive of sparing the rest of the family a care or a financial burden. The analogy is that of Captain Oates sacrificing himself at the South Pole. But in a civilised and compassionate society we do not legislate to encourage such acts. We can respect and even admire them, but we do not promote them via legislation.

---

[33] House of Lords Hansard, 18 July 2014, Cols 830-831

And how in any case is a doctor supposed to be "*satisfied*" that these pressures are not behind a request for 'assisted dying'? A doctor who has known a patient for some considerable time, has regularly seen the patient in his or her home environment and has discussed the request at length with the patient and members of the family may possibly be able to make a knowledge-based judgement in the matter. But, as we have seen, with the majority of doctors unwilling to participate in legalised assistance with suicide and with home visits increasingly rare in community medicine, that sort of doctor-patient relationship is, for large numbers of us, the exception rather than the rule.

Informed Decision

A common feature of 'assisted dying' laws which have been either enacted or proposed is that a person seeking such assistance must be fully informed of the treatments available to relieve his or her condition. So, for example, Oregon's DWDA requires that an applicant for assisted suicide be informed of "*the feasible alternatives including, but not limited to, comfort care, hospice care and pain control*"[34]. Similarly, the bills we have seen at Westminster, including Lord Falconer's latest bill, have required that a person seeking assisted suicide must be "*fully informed of the palliative, hospice and other care which is available*"[35]. Holland's 2001 Termination of Life on Request and Assisted Suicide Act is less specific: it requires that a request for euthanasia or assisted suicide should be "*well considered*" and that the physician "*has informed the patient about the situation he was in and about his prospects*" and that "*the patient holds the conviction that there was no other reasonable solution for the situation he was in*"[36] .

---

[34] DWDA, Section 127.815, sub-section 3.01(c)(E)

[35] HL Bill 69 (Session 2020-21), Clause 3(4)

[36] Termination of Life on Request and Assisted Suicide (Review Procedures) Act 2001, Article 2 (c) and (d)

All this is fair enough, but it raises a number of questions. By whom should this information be imparted? Are we looking at general information from the assessing doctor, who may or may not be up to speed with advances in end-of-life care? Or are we talking about a referral to a specialist in either the patient's terminal illness or palliative medicine in order to explore in depth what can be done for the patient in his or her particular circumstances? The proposed laws we have seen in Britain are silent on these important questions.

Making an informed decision is, in any case, about more than just listening to a briefing. In 2004 the organisation Help the Hospices[37] wrote, in evidence to the Mackay Committee, that:

> "*experience of pain control is radically different from promise of pain control and cessation is almost unimaginable if symptom control has been poor. On this view patients seeking assistance to die without having experienced good symptom control could not be deemed fully informed*"[38].

This raises the question whether there should be what is sometimes called a palliative care filter in any 'assisted dying' legislation - that is to say, that a person requesting physician-assisted suicide should be required to have experience of specialist palliative care before confirming the request. No patient can be compelled to have treatment, though in a situation where a patient is seeking something to which significant risk is attached and which is not regarded as a normal part of clinical care it could be argued that first-hand experience of expert palliative care should be a condition.

---

[37] Now known as Hospice UK

[38] House of Lords Report 86-I (Session 2004-05), Paragraph 258

However, what if such palliative treatment is not available? As a 2015 survey by The Economist Intelligence Unit[39] found, Britain leads the world in the quality of its specialist palliative care. But, as observed in Chapter Four, it is not evenly distributed across the country and, while hospices and specialist palliative care teams in major hospitals are centres of excellence, there can be local gaps or deficiencies in provision at community level. For some, therefore, decisions to take their own lives would be more or less informed than for others.

Quis Custodiet...?

Two thousand years ago the Roman poet Juvenal asked the question "*Quis custodiet ipsos custodes?*", which may be freely translated as 'who is going to keep an eye on the guardians?' It is a question that has relevance in many fields of life, and this is one of them. Even if adequate safeguards can be put in place, what assurance can we have that they will be properly observed by those charged with following them.

The first and obvious step in creating an assurance system is a requirement that there should be arrangements in place for objective post-event audit of the actions that prescribing doctors have taken and appropriate penalties for non-compliance. As noted above, the proposals which have come before the Westminster Parliament have included a requirement that approvals by doctors of requests for lethal drugs should be referred to a judge of the Family Division of the High Court for endorsement before the relevant drugs could be prescribed. That is not, however, an audit system: it is an additional check in the pre-event sequence of events. Moreover, as the Association for Palliative Medicine has argued[40], it could have the perverse effect

---

[39] The 2015 Quality of Death Index, Ranking Palliative Care Across the World, The Economist Intelligence Unit

[40] See Page 145

of encouraging unaccountability by dividing responsibility for the same decision: a doctor who is undecided about a request might be inclined to let it pass in the belief that the Court would act as a long-stop. Moreover, as referral to the Court would take place prior to prescribing, it would provide no means of auditing the post-prescribing phase - for example, whether there was any evidence of pressure having been brought to bear on the patient in the post-approval stage.

The proposals we have seen to date at Westminster require that the Chief Medical Officers of England and Wales should "*monitor the operation of the Act, including compliance with its provisions*"[41]. It is not clear, however, how compliance with the law could be confirmed without a post-event scrutiny system. What is needed is that there should be machinery in place for a light to be shone on how assessments have been made and whether these have been compliant with the law in both the pre-approval and the implementation phases.

As we have seen, such machinery exists in The Netherlands, where doctors who administer euthanasia or assist suicides under the terms of the 2001 Act must report what they have done to regional euthanasia review committees and await their verdict as to whether their actions have complied with the law. As observed in Chapter Five, the rigour with which that review process is conducted is open to question. What is needed, if Britain were ever to have legalised 'assisted dying', is a robust audit system which is able to scrutinise rigorously and impartially how decisions have been reached, to conclude whether the terms of the law have been complied with and, where not, to take appropriate action.

A significant problem here, as noted in Chapter Five, is that all review bodies are, of necessity, made up of human beings, who bring to the task, albeit with the best of intentions, their personal

[41] See, for example, HL Bill 69 (Session 2020-21), Clause 9(1)

views and prejudices. In an area, such as 'assisted dying', where opinion is polarised and there are strongly held views on both sides of the debate, it is very difficult to ensure that bodies which are asked to review such acts are composed of neutral observers or, at least, persons who are not encumbered by political 'baggage' of one sort or another. Such bodies can be expected to attract persons who are sympathetic to legalisation and who, with the best will in the world, may not bring to the task of scrutiny the mindset of challenge and scepticism which all audit activity necessarily involves. Creating an effective audit system would not, therefore, be easy – but it would have to be done.

In Conclusion

Our aim in this chapter has been to show that there is a world of difference between stating seemingly-straightforward conditions, like terminal illness, settled intent and freedom from coercion, and producing safeguards that will stand up to the pressures of the real world and provide serious protection for vulnerable people. There is nothing new about what we have written. The difficulties of devising adequate safeguards for legalised 'assisted dying' have been aired on many occasions. What is surprising is that the advocates of legalisation have failed to respond. In fact, they have in some respects moved backwards. As an example, the late Lord Joffe's 2005 Assisted Dying for the Terminally Ill Private Member Bill included provision for a 'monitoring commission' to audit the management of 'assisted dying' requests, yet this was dropped from subsequent proposals.

Instead of devising more effective safeguards the ‘assisted dying’ lobby has chosen to rely on codes of practice to resolve the problem. They have proposed that Parliament should proceed to legalise assisted suicide on the basis of general criteria, such as terminal illness and freedom from pressure, and that it should be for "*the Secretary of State*" to devise safeguards to give effect to them at a later date.

Thus, Lord Falconer's latest bill states[42] that *"the Secretary of State may issue one or more codes of practice in connection with...the assessment of whether a person has a clear and settled intention to end their own life"*. In other words, the bill is asking Parliament to agree to change the law on assisting suicide on the basis of a handful of broadly-worded criteria (terminal illness, settled intent, freedom from pressure) but it is leaving it to the discretion of the government of the day to decide subsequently how those criteria are to be met.

This raises a constitutional question. Given that the presence of adequate safeguards is of the essence of such legislation (a given which seems to be accepted on both sides of the 'assisted dying' debate), how can Parliament be asked to decide whether the law should be changed to license assistance with suicide unless and until it has seen what the proposed safeguards are and how they would work and has satisfied itself that they are robust enough for the purpose? The answer is that it cannot. In effect, the advocates of legalisation are inviting Parliament to sign a blank cheque.

Some have tried to defend this approach. Take, for example, this statement from Baroness Murphy in the House of Lords:

> *"No legislation on health and social care puts on the face of the Bill the detail of how the Act is to be implemented. We always ask for the professions, and of course the Department of Health involves the professions and the independent professional bodies in trying to deliver a code of practice that is acceptable to the professions which have to deliver the care"*[43]

Of course the detail of legislation need not appear on the face of parliamentary bills and may be relegated to codes of practice. So, for example, the form and sequencing of the paperwork that might be needed in cases of legalised assisted suicide does not necessarily

---

[42] HL Bill 69 (Session 2020-21), Clause 8(1)

[43] House of Lords Hansard, 18 July 2014, Col. 861

have to be approved by Parliament: it can be left to ministerial discretion. But safeguards are not 'detail'. They concern larger questions which are of the essence of legislation such as this - such as, for example, whether and, if so, how the presence of a settled wish can be established and what steps need to be taken to establish freedom from coercion or duress. These are issues consideration of which is central to Parliament's role. Ironically, the bills we have seen in recent years are heavy on bureaucracy - for example, on certification of deaths in cases of assisted suicide - but light on actual safeguards.

We have heard advocates of legalisation argue that their opponents will never be satisfied with any safeguards. There may be an element of truth in this with regard to some of their opponents. But that does not deal with the issue that Parliament is being asked to sign up to a major change to the criminal law without seeing how it would actually work. Anyone contemplating buying a used car would be advised to inspect the service history before, not after, agreeing to the purchase. In the same way Parliament needs to see and consider the safeguards for legalised assisted suicide before, not after, it is invited to consider changing the law. The parliamentary bills we have seen in recent years offer little more than a set of ideals - settled intent, freedom from pressure, capacity to decide. They make little or no provision to govern how those ideals are to be realised in practice. As an analysis of Lord Falconer's 2014 Bill put it:

> "*It is the equivalent of putting up notices on a railway embankment to warn the public against trespassing but not putting any fencing in place to discourage or prevent people from wandering onto the tracks*"[44].

---

[44] "The Assisted Dying Bill: A Critique", published by Living and Dying Well

CHAPTER EIGHT

IN CONCLUSION

ILORA FINLAY AND ROBERT PRESTON

It will be clear from the foregoing chapters that we do not consider an evidence-based case for changing the law has been made. The law as it stands is not perfect - no law is that - but it does the job for which it exists. It sends the clear social message that suicide is not something to be encouraged or assisted. It has the teeth to cause anyone minded to assist another person's suicide to think very carefully indeed before proceeding. And it has, built-into it, discretion to deal sensitively with genuinely compassionate acts of assistance. In these circumstances it is hardly surprising that the incidence of assisting suicide is very small and that the few cases that do occur tend to be those where the circumstances have been exceptional and where prosecution is not required in the public interest. What has been proposed is something very different – the licensing of assistance with suicide in advance and for specific groups of people who appear to meet certain broadly-defined criteria.

In legislative terms an 'assisted dying' law may look like a small adjustment of the law. But its effect would be huge. It would license the deliberate bringing about of the deaths of individuals in certain perceived circumstances. That does not necessarily mean that such a change should not be made, but it does mean that there must be clear evidence that the existing law, which prohibits such actions, is in need of change and that what would be put in its place would be better – and, above all, would protect vulnerable people. In our view not only does that evidence not exist but there is serious evidence to the contrary.

Let us suppose, however, that a convincing case for changing the law were to be made. Would that alter the situation as regards legalisation? In that event two requirements would remain to be met. One is that any legislation would have to include safeguards robust enough to protect vulnerable people from harm. That has not been done to date. The proposals we have seen, both north and south of the English-Scottish border, come nowhere near to meeting the stringent safety requirements needed for a change in the law of such gravity.

The seeker of assisted suicide who steps out of the pages of the parliamentary bills which have been tabled in London and Edinburgh is the stereotypical no-nonsense and strong-willed individual who is set on ending his or her life, has thought long and hard about the decision and is not in any way vulnerable. The role allocated to the doctor is one of running the rule over what is assumed to be a well-considered request rather than bringing any kind of serious challenge to it. The underlying picture which these proposals paint is of patients who know exactly what they are doing and of doctors who know them well and are able to make social as well as medical judgements about them without difficulty. It is impossible to read these bills without feeling that they have been written for a particular constituency rather than with the interests of society as a whole in mind.

Any future proposals for legal change need to incorporate real-world safeguards whose implications have been thought through and which make clear how they would work in practice. In Chapter Seven we have highlighted the serious deficiencies in what so far have been called safeguards and in some cases we have suggested how these might be made more effective. This is serious work and the 'assisted dying' lobby needs to get to grips with it and to produce rigorous safeguards that will stand up to the pressures of terminal illness, medical practice and complex family dynamics. The broadly-worded criteria which have featured in Private Member bills to date simply will not suffice.

The second requirement is to address the question: who should be assessing requests for 'assisted dying' and deciding the outcome? There are serious objections to loading these tasks onto the shoulders of hard-pressed clinicians, many of whom have considerable reservations about such practices and would be unwilling to have anything to do with them. As we have argued above, doctors may have a role to play in providing expert advice on strictly medical aspects of a request for 'assisted dying', but they are in no position to be decision-makers over whether such a request should be granted. Gathering and weighing evidence and decision-making should be the responsibility of the High Court – and of the Court alone.

These are challenging requirements which have not been addressed, but they must be if Parliament is to be asked yet again to consider changing the law. We are dealing here with a complex and emotive subject. It is also a matter which has the potential to do serious harm, both to individuals and to the social fabric, if not handled with care. The campaigning which has been taking place for legal change to date has been conducted in a superficial manner, relying on soundbites, opinion polling and celebrity endorsements. This is wholly insufficient for a matter of such gravity.